Cancer in pregnancy, although thankfully a relatively uncommon occurrence, presents physicians and their patients with a major dilemma. The urge to use the highest tolerable doses of chemotherapy, high doses of irradiation and surgery has to be weighed carefully against their risks to the unborn baby. This book is the very first to attempt to quantify these risks and to provide physicians with a core of knowledge that will be very relevant to making sound clinical decisions in the face of sometimes conflicting interests. The volume evaluates the results of the Motherisk Program, which was set up specifically to address this problem, and reviews maternal and fetal outcomes from a sizeable database of the most common cases of cancer in pregnancy. In reviewing this program and the experience of others in this area, this volume sets out to create a clinically relevant tool for oncologists, obstetrician–gynecologists, perinatologists and neonatologists.

CANCER IN PREGNANCY:
MATERNAL AND FETAL RISKS

CANCER IN PREGNANCY: MATERNAL AND FETAL RISKS

Edited by

G. KOREN
*Department of Pediatrics, The Hospital for Sick Children,
University of Toronto, Canada*

M. LISHNER
*Department of Medicine, Sapir Medical Center, Kefan Saba,
Sackler School of Medicine, Tel Aviv University, Israel*

D. FARINE
*Department of Obstetrics and Gynecology, Division of
Maternal–Fetal Medicine, Mount Sinai Hospital, University
of Toronto, Canada*

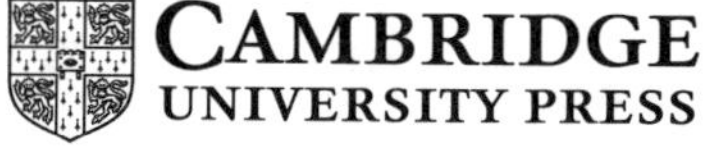

CAMBRIDGE
UNIVERSITY PRESS

Published by the Press Syndicate of the University of Cambridge
The Pitt Building, Trumpington Street, Cambridge CB2 1RP
40 West 20th Street, New York, NY 10011–4211, USA
10 Stamford Road, Oakleigh, Melbourne 3166, Australia

© Cambridge University Press 1996

First published 1996

Printed in Great Britain at the University Press, Cambridge

A catalogue record for this book is available from the British Library

Library of Congress cataloguing in publication data available

ISBN 0 521 47176 1 hardback

Contents

Part III: Fetal effects of cancer and its treatment

Preface

Cancer is the second leading cause of death in women during the reproductive years, and its occurrence in pregnancy is between 0.07% and 0.1%.

The relative rare occurrence of cancer during pregnancy precludes the conduct of large prospective studies to examine diagnostic, management and outcome issues. However, when cancer occurs during gestation, it creates immense pressure on the pregnant patient, her family and her physicians. The urge to use the highest tolerable doses of chemotherapy, high doses of irradiation and surgery have to be carefully weighted against their potential risks to the unborn baby. This often may result in maternal fetal conflicts.

In order for the woman and her family to arrive at the optimal personal decision, which will drive the medical management, one has to ensure that the family is optimally informed. This is extremely difficult when information is sparse or missing, as is the case in many forms of cancer in pregnancy.

Since the inception of the Motherisk Program in 1985, we have become painfully aware of the lack of data to guide the difficult decisions surrounding the management of cancer in pregnancy. To try to address this unacceptable gap, we commenced our case control studies using the Princess Margaret Hospital database which had accumulated in its thirty years of existence over 300 cases of cancer in pregnancy.

In parallel lines of investigation we have also attempted to critically review the world experience on issues such as irradiation of cancer chemotherapy, as well as using *in vitro* models to study the role of the placenta in fetal carcinogenesis.

Much of the data produced by The Motherisk study group and included in this volume have been published in peer reviewed journals in North

America and Europe over the last five years. Some of it, however, is presented here for the first time.

We hope that assembling this effort into one volume and adding to it critical review of related issues (e.g. effects of specific drugs), we would create a clinically relevant tool for oncologists, obstetrician–gynecologists, perinatologists, neonatologists, as well as cancer biologists and other scientists dealing with cancer research.

The editors are indebted to the Department of Biostatistics of The Princess Margaret Hospital and to Mrs Niki Balamatsis of The Division of Clinical Pharmacology at The Hospital for Sick Children for preparation of this manuscript.

Gideon Koren, MD
Michael Lishner, MD
Dan Farine, MD
Toronto and Tel Aviv
June 1995

Contributors

Y. Bentur
Senior Lecturer, Department of Medicine, Technion, Israel, Israel Poison Information Center, Haifa 31096, Israel.

P. Degendorfer
Department of Statistics, Princess Margaret Hospital, Toronto, Ontario, Canada.

L. Derewlany
Assistant Professor of Pediatrics, Division of Clinical Pharmacology/ Toxicology, The Hospital for Sick Children, and University of Toronto, Ontario, Canada.

Y. Ezra
Department of Obstetrics and Gynecology, Hadassah Einkerem Hospital, Hebrew University, Jerusalem, Israel.

D. Farine
Associate Professor of Obstetrics and Gynecology, Department of Obstetrics and Gynecology, Division of Maternal Fetal Medicine, Mount Sinai Hospital, University of Toronto, Toronto, Ontario, Canada.

E. N. Kelly
Assistant Professor of Pediatrics, Department of Pediatrics, Division of Neonatology, Mount Sinai Hospital, University of Toronto, Toronto, Ontario, Canada.

G. Koren
Professor of Pediatrics, Pharmacology, Pharmacy and Medicine, The Motherisk Program, Division of Clinical Pharmacology/Toxicology, Department of Pediatrics, The Hospital for Sick Children and The University of Toronto, Toronto, Ontario, Canada.

M. Lishner
Department of Medicine, Sapir Medical Center, Kefar Saba, Israel, and Tel Aviv University, Israel.

P. McParland
National Maternity Hospital, Holles Street, Dublin, Ireland.

K. Panter
Department of Obstetrics and Gynecology, Division of Maternal–Fetal Medicine, Toronto, Ontario, Canada.

T. Panzarella
Department of Statistics, Princess Margaret Hospital, Toronto, Ontario, Canada.

A. Pastuszak
The Motherisk Program, Division of Clinical Pharmacology/Toxicology, The Hospital for Sick Children, Toronto, Ontario, Canada.

M. Ravid
Professor of Medicine, Sapir Medical Center, Kefan Saba, Israel and Sackler School of Medicine, Tel Aviv University, Israel.

I. B. Rosen
Professor of Surgery, University of Toronto, Co-Director Head and Neck Program, Mount Sinai Hospital, Consultant in Surgery, Princess Margaret Hospital, Toronto, Ontario, Canada.

G. Ryan
National Maternity Hospital, Holles Street, Dublin, Ireland.

S. B. Sutcliffe
Professor of Radiology and President, Princess Margaret Hospital, Toronto, Ontario, Canada.

D. Zemlickis
The Motherisk Program, Division of Clinical Pharmacology/Toxicology, Department of Pediatrics, The Hospital for Sick Children, Toronto, Ontario, Canada.

Part I

Introduction

1
Cancer in pregnancy: identification of unanswered questions on maternal and fetal risks

G. KOREN, M. LISHNER AND D. ZEMLICKIS

When cancer occurs in pregnancy, there is almost always a conflict between optimal maternal therapy and fetal well-being. Consequently, either maternal or fetal health, or both, may be compromised.

Very sparse data exist on maternal outcome after cancer treatment in pregnancy. In addition, the literature on fetal outcome following maternal cancer is composed mainly of case reports. As a result, guidelines for therapy are based on very limited data, and often on few reported cases.

In this review, we analyze the available data regarding the impact of pregnancy on the course of cancer and the effects of the malignant process and its treatment on both the mother and her fetus. The purpose of this analysis is to identify areas where available data may allow clear conclusions as well as crystallization of questions which should have to be answered by future research.

Cancer in pregnancy

Cancer is the second most common cause of death during the reproductive years, complicating approximately 1/1000 pregnancies[1]. The most common malignancies associated with pregnancy include breast, cervix, leukemia, lymphoma, melanoma, thyroid, ovary, and colon. Because of the current trend for many women to delay child-bearing, the association of these malignancies with pregnancy is likely to increase. In previous decades, pregnancy was discouraged in patients with a history of cancer. However, in the current era such pregnancies are supported with more optimism. Conception in a patient over the age of 35, or in any patient believed to have diminished child-bearing potential, is considered a "valued pregnancy".

The discovery of cancer during pregnancy presents an extreme stress to both patient and physician. Because optimization of both maternal and fetal outcomes may be impossible, compromise in the case of either mother or baby may be necessary. Clear guidelines for the management of these patients are essential, however, because the number of reported cases of pregnancy complicated by cancer is small and current management strategies are based on anecdotal reports, often presenting conflicting information[1].

One of the most common types of cancer during pregnancy is carcinoma of the breast. This cancer complicates 1/3000 pregnancies, representing 3% of all breast cancers[2]. Reports in the literature are limited to small numbers of patients, suggesting that stage for stage, the prognosis is the same for pregnant and nonpregnant patients. However, because pregnant patients often present with more advanced disease, they tend to have worse prognoses than nonpregnant patients of the same age[3]. While the outcome appears to be worse in patients below the age of 30 years[3] and in those diagnosed in the second half of pregnancy[4], the reasons for these tendencies are unknown.

The effect of the altered hormonal environment of pregnancy on the growth of breast tumors is the subject of controversy, with some authors reporting a more rapid progression of disease in pregnancy, while others report no such difference[3]. Several important questions remain unanswered. Is it ever safe to delay treatment because of the pregnancy? Is it safe to administer chemotherapy or radiation after the first trimester? Does the tumor progress more rapidly during pregnancy[2,3,5]? Should the pregnancy be terminated early? When and how should the baby be delivered?

Lymphomas are relatively common malignancies during the reproductive years. At the time of initial diagnosis or relapse of Hodgkin's disease, one-third of premenopausal patients are pregnant or have delivered within 2 years[6]. Sutcliffe and Chapman[7] suggested that "pregnancy does not affect the course of Hodgkin's disease and the disease does not affect the course of the pregnancy"; however, this conclusion was based on a review of the literature published prior to 1977. The treatment of the lymphomas depends on accurate staging, which requires such procedures as lymphangiogram, intravenous pyelography (IVP), computed tomography scans, and staging laparotomy[7-9] exposing the fetus to the potential risks of radiation and xenobiotics. As those patients with the earliest disease have the greatest chance of cure, it is crucial that accurate staging be performed. As in the case of breast cancer, a variety of questions remain unanswered: should therapy be delayed to optimize fetal outcome or instituted immediately to maximize the mother's chance of cure?

The acute leukemias are very rare during pregnancy, suggesting that fertility may be diminished in these patients[10,11]. Although there is no evidence to date indicating that either the acute or chronic leukemias are altered by a coexisting pregnancy[12], the number of patients studied has been very small. Since acute leukemias are highly malignant but potentially curable, the best available regimen should be used in the woman presenting in the first trimester immediately following decision regarding the continuation of the pregnancy. Many reports exist of delivery of normal babies to women despite intensive treatment in subsequent trimesters[13,14].

Papillary adenocarcinoma of the thyroid, the most common of the thyroid neoplasms, has a peak age distribution in women of 30 to 34 years. The actual incidence of thyroid cancer during pregnancy is unknown. In patients under the age of 49, 90 to 95% survive 15 years[15,16]. Retrospective reviews suggest that pregnancy has a negligible effect on tumor progression[17,18]. However, treatment of this cancer is altered by the presence of a pregnancy: tumor ablation with radioactive iodine is contraindicated during pregnancy owing to adverse fetal effects, and, in patients with early disease, this therapy is offered postpartum.

In patients with more advanced disease, surgical excision of the tumor during pregnancy followed postpartum by radiotherapy is the treatment of choice[19]. In one study, radical neck dissection was followed by miscarriage in three of five patients[20].

Malignant melanoma is diagnosed in two to three of every 1000 pregnancies[21,22], and 30 to 35% of melanoma patients are women of reproductive age. Estrogen receptor protein has been isolated in melanoma cells, suggesting the possibility that this tumor may be hormone dependent[23]. However, the effect of pregnancy on the behavior of existing melanomas is in dispute because partial and complete postpartum regressions of melanomas have been reported[24–26]. Some authors report no effect of pregnancy on survival in patients with melanoma, whereas others report diminished survival in comparison with nonpregnant patients[27,28]. Here too, most reports are based on small numbers of patients.

Ovarian cancer is the fourth leading cause of all cancer deaths. However, it is so rarely diagnosed during pregnancy that solid management guidelines are lacking and it is unknown if pregnancy *per se* alters the natural history of the tumor. Experience in the nonpregnant state remains the basis for management[29].

Carcinoma of the cervix is the malignancy most commonly associated with pregnancy[30,31]. The Pap smear reveals abnormal cytology in 3% of pregnant patients with 4% of these due to invasive cancer. One out of every 30 cases of invasive cervical cancer occurs during pregnancy, complicating

1/1250 pregnancies. There is considerable controversy regarding the effect of pregnancy on the progression of cervical tumors. Findings from several studies suggest that the prognosis is poorer when there is an associated pregnancy, while others show no such detrimental effect[32,33]. Nisker and Shubert[33] reported an increased incidence of positive IB disease, as compared to nonpregnant patients. They also noted an increased risk of complications following radiation therapy and a lower 5-year survival rate in pregnant patients. Current unresolved issues include the following. Is there any benefit to delivery by cesarean section rather than vaginal delivery? What facts are needed for patients to consider termination of pregnancy? Should labor be induced? If so, at what gestational age should labor be induced? Should the pregnancy affect the decision to treat with surgery versus radiation?

Risks to the fetus

In discussing potential risk to the fetus associated with maternal cancer, one should consider the following:
1. The effect of chemotherapy and radiation on the developing fetus;
2. The effect of maternal anesthesia and surgery on the fetus;
3. The effect of maternal illness on fetal well-being.

Chemotherapy and radiation

With the establishment of sensitive analytical methods for measurement of drug levels in body fluids, it has become apparent that almost all xenobiotics are capable of crossing the placenta. Although cancer chemotherapy drugs belong to a variety of pharmacological groups, their common denominator is their ability to adversely affect cell division. Thus, the very qualities which make such compounds desirable for cancer therapy make them detrimental to the developing embryo. Animal studies reveal that almost all antineoplastic agents are teratogenic[34], and the sensitive period corresponds to the time of organogenesis (the first trimester in human pregnancy).

Evidence of teratogenic potential in humans is derived from case reports or small series. These total less than 250 cases as of 1987[34]. The American National Cancer Institute has established a registry of patients exposed to cancer chemotherapy during gestation. By 1987, 204 cases had been filed[35]. The generalizability of findings is highly tenuous because the denominator, or total number of such exposures, is not known. It can be argued, for example, that clinicians choose to report only adverse outcomes, thus overrepresenting teratogenic potential of chemotherapy. Conversely, it may be argued that a normal outcome is deemed important enough to be reported[36].

Administration of chemotherapy in the first trimester of pregnancy exposes the embryo during embryogenesis to toxicity that may manifest an embryonic death or gross malformations[37]. Approximately 10% of fetuses exposed to cytotoxic drugs during the first trimester of pregnancy exhibit major malformations[38,39] compared to a rate of 1 to 3% in the general population. Among the cytotoxic agents, only aminopterin, a folic acid antagonist which is not used any more, has been shown to cause increased malformation rates[40]. There are at least 16 documented cases of teratogenic effect of the drug when used alone[34]. Methotrexate, a drug closely related to aminopterin was associated with birth defects in at least three cases but the rate of their occurrence is lower[34]. Their use should be avoided in the first trimester of pregnancy. Based on collection of case reports from the literature, the estimated relative risk for malformation was reported to be 1:9 for busulfan, 1:6 for cyclophosphamide, and 1:2 for chlorambucil[41]. Single reports exist on congenital malformation with the use of 5 flurouracil[40] and azothiomine[41] and arabinosyl cytosine[42,43]. Antibiotics (anthracyclines, bleomycin) and vinca alkaloids (vincristine, vinblastine) were not reported to cause malformation when administered during the first trimester[34].

There are only a few case reports regarding the use of single, other antineoplastics during early pregnancy. Although no association between the use of these drugs and congenital malformation was noted, their teratogenic risk cannot be estimated.

In a recent review of the literature, Doll *et al*[44] found that the rate of fetal malformation from combination of drugs in the first trimester is only slightly higher than observed with single agents; six (25%) of 24 cases versus 24 (17%) of 139 cases.

Based on small series and case reports, exposure to chemotherapy after the first trimester does not appear to pose an increased teratogenic risk. This observation is expected because embryogenesis of somatic organs is completed by 12 weeks. Brain development, by contrast, is a lengthier process. Consequently, xenobiotics are known to affect central nervous system development adversely in the second and third trimesters (e.g. methyl mercury, lead, and PCBs)[45–47].

Only one study is known to have measured long-term developmental outcome specifically. Aviles and Niz[48] examined 17 offspring of women with acute leukemia during pregnancy. Neurological, intellectual and visual–motor–perceptual assessments were administered to the offspring who ranged in age from 4 to 22 years, and to siblings and unrelated controls. No differences were detected between the groups. Interpretation of the findings are constrained by the lack of presentation of data, the question as to whether the children were assessed "blind", and the use of a cross-sectional rather than a longitudinal design. Moreover, the inclusion in the sample of children whose mothers did not receive chemotherapy permits conclusions about the consequences of the disease, but it limits the understanding of the effects of chemotherapy. Notwithstanding the limitations, this study is important as the only existing examination of developmental outcome following exposure *in utero* to cytotoxic therapy. The general impression, based on case reports, is that chemotherapy does not have a major impact on later development. However, studies of the developmental teratogenicity of such environmental toxins as lead demonstrate that complex study designs are needed to detect small, but clinically relevant effects.

Other long-term adverse effects of *in utero* exposure to chemotherapy also must be considered. Recently in Toronto, a case of congenital malformation[49] was described in a child exposed *in utero* to cyclophosphamide for the treatment of maternal leukemia. The same child later developed both neuroblastoma and thyroid carcinoma. Of special interest is the fact that his twin sister is normal, suggesting the possibility of pharmacogenetic differences in metabolism of cyclophosphamide. Another example of the long-term teratogenic effects of *in utero* exposure to toxins is the occurrence of clear cell vaginal carcinoma in women exposed *in utero* to diethylstilbestrol[50].

Cancer chemotherapeutic agents are known to affect the fetal hematopoetic system. For example, cytopenia at birth has been described by a number of authors. However, because case reports yield little opportunity for statistical comparisons, the real risk of neonatal cytopenia following transplacental transfer of chemotherapeutic agents is unknown. Recently, Reynoso *et al*[49] surveyed existing case reports and integrated the findings with their own experience at the Toronto Leukemia Study Group. From this data base, they estimated that about one-third of all infants exposed *in utero* to chemotherapy will experience pancytopenia at birth[49].

Maternal exposure to radiation, either for diagnostic or therapeutic reasons, may increase fetal risks. To date, it is believed that fetal exposure to less than 0.05 Gy does not increase the teratogenic risk. In most diagnostic procedures, the cumulative exposure does not reach this dose level, even when the maternal abdomen is not shielded. However, the diagnosis of maternal cancer is often complicated and may require a battery of radio-diagnostic tests whose cumulative radiation dose may potentially exceed the 0.1 Gy level. In the case of radiation therapy, substantially higher dose levels are involved, and these have been shown unequivocally to result in fetal damage, mainly to the brain, as evidenced by microcephaly and developmental delay[51].

Surgery

Surgery is conducted either to diagnose or to eradicate cancer. In both instances, the fetus is exposed to the potential risks from the transplacental effects of anesthetic agents, as well as to complications of maternal surgery. There are large published studies which establish the safety during pregnancy of the most commonly used anesthetic agents, including nitrous oxide, enflurane, barbiturates, and narcotics[34]. However, intraoperative complications, such as hypoxia, hypotension, hypovolemia, and decreased utero-placental perfusion secondary to prolonged maintenance in the supine position, as well as postoperative morbidity in the form of fever, infection, poor nutritional intake, or even pulmonary embolus, do threaten fetal well-being[44].

Maternal well-being

The cancer patient has an increased tendency to suffer febrile illness from infectious sources, drug fever, and/or the tumor *per se*. Numerous animal studies have shown a correlation between maternal hyperthermia and increased incidence of abortions and malformations, most notably microcephaly, microphthalmia, and skeletal defects[52–57]. Germain[58] found a threshold of 2.5 °C increase in core temperature for 1 hour was sufficient to induce malformations in rats, whereas increases in temperature of less than 2 °C were not found to be teratogenic. The sensitive period for teratogenesis was the era of gastrulation.

The relationship between hyperthermia and malformations in humans is less well defined. One obvious difficulty is the separation of the effects of fever from those of its cause, such as viral illness[59]. Many human studies do support the hypothesis that maternal febrile illness in early pregnancy is teratogenic, with neural tube defects and microphthalmia the most commonly noted anomalies. However, causal association has not been established[59–66].

Proper maternal nutrition is important for optimal neonatal and maternal outcome. However, the degree of maternal undernutrition which can be tolerated by the fetus without adverse effects has not been established. Studies with animals have indicated that severe maternal undernutrition can result in stillbirths and increased perinatal mortality[67]. However, retrospective analysis of human data obtained during historical periods of starvation have revealed little or no adverse fetal effects[68].

Review of perinatal morbidity and mortality following severe food deprivation in the Netherlands during World War II revealed a mean decrease in birth weight of 8 oz, but no increase in congenital malformations or perinatal mortality[69]. Analysis of military screening examinations on all Dutch males at age 19 failed to disclose any difference in IQ score between boys whose mothers were starved during pregnancy and the general male population[70]. Elsewhere, studies have indicated adverse fetal effects following maternal malnutrition[71–74]. Additionally, studies have suggested that maternal ketoacidosis, as encountered in dehydration or severe weight loss, is potentially detrimental to fetal develpment[75,76].

Based on the above, it is evident that detriments in maternal well-being, such as malnutrition and fever, may pose additional risks to the developing embryo–fetus. These conditions are encountered more frequently in the cancer patient.

In summary, many questions regarding the management and outcome of the pregnant woman who develops a malignant disease and its impact on the fetus remain unanswered. The existence of pregnancy in the patient with cancer may have both a direct (e.g., hormonal changes) and indirect impacts on the course and management of the disease. This includes delay in diagnostic workup and treatment, choice of therapy, psychological stress, etc. In addition, chemotherapy and its associated side effects may bear teratogenic potential as well as long-term adverse effects such as developmental disturbances, infertility or malignancies.

The decision-making is complex due to physiological, moral, and ethical aspects of this extremely stressful situation. It is further complicated by the existence of only sparse data on both maternal and fetal outcome. Large, multicenter collaborative studies are needed to evaluate both the effects of pregnancy on the course of cancer and that of the malignant process and its treatment on the mother and her offspring. Such studies will allow the development of rational management policies.

References

1. Allen HH, Nisker JA: *Cancer in Pregnancy*. 1986, p. 3, Futura Publishing Company Inc., Mt. Kisco, New York.
2. Parente JT, Amsel M, Lerner R *et al*: Breast cancer associated with pregnancy. *Obstet Gynecol* 1988; 71: 861.

3. Bush H, McCredie JA: Carcinoma of the breast during pregnancy and lactation. In *Cancer in Pregnancy* (Allen H, Nisker AJ eds.) 1986, p. 91, Futura Publishing Company, Inc., Mt. Kisco, New York.

4. Peters MV, Meakin JW: The influence of pregnancy in carcinoma of the breast. In *Progress in Clinical Cancer* (Ariel IM ed.) 1965, vol. 1, p. 471, Grune and Stratton, New York.

5. Peters MV: Effect of pregnancy in breast cancer. In *Prognostic Factors in Breast Cancer* (Forrest APM, Kunkler PB eds.) 1968, p. 65, Williams and Wilkins, Baltimore.

6. Chapman RM, Sutcliffe SB, Malpas JS: Cytotoxic-induced ovarian failure in women with Hodgkin's disease: I. Hormone function. *JAMA* 1979; 242: 1877.

7. Sutcliffe SB, Chapman RM: Lymphomas and leukemias. In *Cancer in Pregnancy* (Allen HH, Nisker JA ed.) 1986, p. 135, Futura, Mt. Kisco, New York.

8. Kaplan HS: Clinical evaluation. In *Hodgkin's Disease*, (Kaplan HS. 2nd edn.) 1980, p. 116, Harvard University Press, Cambridge.

9. Sutcliffe SB, Timothy AR, Lister TA: Staging in Hodgkin's disease. *Clin Haematol* 1979; 8: 593.

10. McClain CR Jr.: Leukemia in pregnancy. *Clin Obstet Gynecol* 1974; 17: 185.

11. Hoover BA, Schumacher HR: Acute leukemia in pregnancy. *Am J Obstet Gynecol* 1966; 96: 316.

12. Nicholson HO: Leukemia and pregnancy. A report of five cases and discussion of management. *J Obstet Gynecol Br Commonw* 1968; 75: 517.

13. Fassas A, Kartalis G, Klearchou N *et al*: Chemotherapy for acute leukemia during pregnancy. *Nour Rev Fr Hematol* 1984; 26: 19.

14. Catanzarite JA, Ferguson JE: Acute leukemia and pregnancy. A review of management outcome: 1972–1982. *Obstet Gynecol Surv* 1984; 39: 663.

15. Cady B, Sedgwick CE, Meissner WA *et al*: Changing clinical, pathologic, therapeutic and survival patterns in differentiated thyroid carcinoma. *Ann Surg* 1976; 184: 541.

16. Cady B, Sedgwick CE, Meissner WA *et al*: Risk factor analysis in differentiated thyroid. *Cancer* 1979; 43: 810.

17. Hill CS, Clark RL, Wolf M: The effect of subsequent pregnancy on patients with thyroid carcinoma. *Surg Gynecol Obstet* 1966; 122: 1219.

18. Donegan WL: Cancer and pregnancy. *Cancer* 1983; 33: 194.

19. Stuart GCE, Temple WJ: Thyroid cancer in pregnancy. In *Cancer in Pregnancy* (Allen HH, Nisker JA. ed.) 1986, p. 3, Futura, Mt. Kisco, New York.

20. Cunningham MP, Slaughter DP: Surgical treatment of disease of the thyroid gland in pregnancy. *Surg Gynecol Obstet* 1970; 131: 486.

21. Smith RS, Randall P: Melanoma during pregnancy. *Obstet Gynecol* 1969; 34: 825.

22. Deleted in press.

23. Fisher RI, Neifeld JP, Lippman ME: Oestrogen receptors in human malignant melanoma. *Lancet* 1976; ii: 337.

24. Sumner WC: Spontaneous regression of melanoma: report of a case. *Cancer* 1953; 6: 1040.

25. Allen AC: A reorientation on the histogenesis and clinical significance of cutaneous nevi and melanomas. *Cancer* 1949; 2: 28.

26. Breslow A: Thickness, cross-sectional areas, and depth of invasion in the prognosis of cutaneous melanoma. *Ann Surg* 1970; 172: 902.

27. Tapeznikov NN, Khasanov SR, Lavorskii, VV: Melanoma of the skin and pregnancy. *Vopr-Oncol* 1987; 33: 40.
28. Reintgen SM: Malignant melanoma and pregnancy. *Cancer* 1985; 55: 1340.
29. Halmo SD, Nisker JA, Allen HH: Primary ovarian cancer in pregnancy. In *Cancer in Pregnancy* (Allen HH, Nisker JA. eds.) p. 269, 1986, Futura Publishing Company Inc., Mt. Kisco, New York.
30. Nieminen N, Remes N: Malignancy during pregnancy. *Acta Obst. Gynecol. Scand.* 1970; 49: 315.
31. Barber HR, Brunschwig A: Gynecologic cancer complicating pregnancy. *Am. J. Obstet Gynecol* 1963; 85: 156.
32. Hacker NF, Berek JS, Lagasse LD *et al*: Carcinoma of the cervix associated with pregnancy. *Obstet Gynecol* 1982; 59: 235.
33. Nisker JA, Shubert M: Stage IB cervical carcinoma and pregnancy: report of 49 cases. *Am J Obstet Gynecol* 1983; 145: 203.
34. Schardein JL: Cancer chemotherapeutic agents. In *Chemically Induced Birth Defects* (Schardein JL. ed.) 1985, p. 467, Marcel Dekker Inc., NY and Basel.
35. The First International Conference of Teratogen Information Services, Boston, MA, April 25, 1988.
36. Mulrihill JJ, McKeen EA, Rosner F *et al*: Pregnancy outcome in cancer patients. Experience in a large cooperative group. *Cancer* 1987; 60: 1143.
37. Sutcliffe SB: Treatment of neoplastic disease during pregnancy: maternal and fetal effects. *Clin Invest Med* 1985; 8: 333.
38. Nicholson HO: Cytotoxic drugs in pregnancy. Review of reported cases. *J Obstet Gynecol Br Commonw* 1968; 75: 307.
39. Warkany J: Aminopterin and methotrexate. Folic acid deficiency. *Teratology* 1978; 17: 353.
40. Stephens JD, Globus MS, Miller TR *et al*: Multiple congenital anomalies in a fetus exposed to 5 Fluroracil during the first trimester. *Am J Obstet Gynecol*, 1980; 137: 747.
41. Williamson RA, Karp LE: Azathioprine teratogenicity: review of the literature and case report. *Obstet Gynecol* 1981; 58: 247.
42. Wagner VM, Hill JS, Weaver D *et al*: Congenital abnormalities in a baby born to cytarabine treated mother. *Lancet* 1980; ii: 98.
43. Schafer AI: Teratogenic effects of antileukemic chemotherapy. *Arch Intern Med* 1981; 141: 514.
44. Doll DC, Ringenberg QS, Yarbo JW: Management of cancer during pregnancy. *Arch Int Med* 1988; 14: 2058.
45. Koren G: Human teratogens. In *Maternal Fetal Toxicology: Clinician's Guide.* (Koren, G. ed.) 1990, Marcel Dekker, New York.
46. Rogan WJ, Gladen BC, Hung KL: Congenital poisoning by polychlorinated biphenyls and their contaminants in Taiwan. *Science* 1988; 241: 334.
47. Harada M: Congenital Minamata disease: intrauterine methylmercury poisoning. *Teratology* 1978; 18: 285.
48. Aviles A, Niz J: Long-term follow-up of children born to mothers with acute leukemia during pregnancy. *Med Pediatr Oncol* 1988; 16: 3.
49. Reynoso EE, Shepherd FA, Messner HA *et al*: Acute leukemia during pregnancy: the Toronto Leukemia Study Group experience with long-term follow-up of children exposed *in utero* to chemotherapeutic agents. *J Clin Oncol* 1987; 5: 1098.
50. Herbst AL, Ulfedert H, Poskanzer DC: Adenocarcinoma of the vagina. Association of maternal stilbestrol therapy with tumor appearance in young

women. *N Engl J Med* 1971; 248: 878.
51. National Council on Radiation Protection and Measurements. Medical radiation exposure of pregnant and potentially pregnant women. *NCRP Report No. 54 32*, 1979.
52. Edwards MJ: Congenital defects in guinea pigs following induced hyperthermia during gestation. *Arch Pathol* 1967; 84: 42.
53. Edwards MJ: Congenital defects in guinea pigs: fetal resorptions, abortions and malformations following induced hyperthermia during early gestation. *Teratology* 1969a; 2: 313.
54. Blishen BR, Carroll WK, Moore C: The 1981 socioeconomic index for occupations in Canada. *Can Rev Sociol Anthropol* 1987; 24: 465.
55. Webster WS, Germain MA, Edwards MJ: The induction of microphthalmia, encephalocele and other head defects following hyperthermia during the gastrulation process in the rat. *Teratology* 1985; 16: 73.
56. Kilham FVH: Exencephaly in fetal hamsters following exposure to hyperthermia. *Teratology* 1976; 14: 323.
57. Umpierre CC, Bukelow WR: Environmental heat stress effects in the hamster. *Teratology* 1977; 16: 155.
58. Germain MA, Webster WS, Edwards MJ: Hyperthermia as a teratogen: parameters determining hyperthermia-induced head defects in the rat. *Teratology* 1985; 31: 265.
59. Workany J: Teratogen update: hyperthermia. *Teratology* 1986; 33: 365.
60. Edwards MJ: Influenza, hyperthermia, and congenital malformations. *Lancet* 1972; i: 320.
61. Miller P, Smith DW, Spherd TH: Maternal hyperthermia as a possible cause for anencephaly. *Lancet* 1978; i: 519.
62. Chance PF, Smith DW: Hyperthermia and meningomyelocele and anencephaly. *Lancet* 1978; i: 769.
63. Layde PM, Edmonds LD, Erickson JD: Maternal fever and neural tube defects. *Teratology* 1980; 21: 105.
64. James WH: Hyperthermia and meningomyelocele and anencephaly. (Letter). *Lancet* 1978; i: 770.
65. Kleinebrecht J, Michaelis H, Michaelis J *et al:* Fever in pregnancy and congenital anomalies. (Letter). *Lancet* 1979; i: 1043.
66. Clarren SK, Smith DW, Harvey MA: Hyperthermia: a prospective evaluation of a possible teratogenic agent in man. *J Pediatr* 1979; 95: 81.
67. Hechner AJ: Interaction of prenatal starvation and dexamethasone treatment on lung development in newborn guinea pigs. *Am Rev Respir Dis* 1987; 135: 991.
68. Pritchard JA, MacDonald PC, Gant NF: *Williams Obstetrics*, 17th edn. 1985, Appleton-Century-Crofts, Norwalk, CT.
69. Smith CA: Effects of maternal undernutrition upon the newborn infant in Holland (1944–1945). *J Pediatr* 1947; 30: 229.
70. Stein Z, Sussur M, Saenger G *et al:* Nutrition and mental performance. *Science* 1972; 178: 708.
71. Metcoff S, Castillae JP, Crosby W: Maternal nutrition and fetal outcome. *Am. J. Clin Nutr* 1981; 34 (supp. 4): 708.
72. Rosso P: Prenatal nutrition and fetal growth and development. *Pediatr Ann* 1981; 10: 21.
73. Brown JE, Jacobson HN, Askue LH: Influence of pregnancy weight gain on the size of infants born to underweight women. *Obstet Gynecol* 1981; 57: 13.

74. Edwards LE, Alton IR, Barrada MI *et al*: Pregnancy in the underweight
    woman: course, outcome and growth patterns of infant. *Am J Obstet Gynecol*
    1979; 135: 297.
75. Churchill JA, Benendex HW: Intelligence of children whose mothers had
    acetonuria during pregnancy. In *Perinatal Factors Affecting Human
    Development*, 1969, Pan American Sanitary Bureau, Washington.
76. Naeyl RL, Chez RA: Effects of maternal acetonuria and low pregnancy
    weight gain on children's psychomotor development. *Am J Obstet Gynecol*
    1981; 139: 189.

2

The pregnant patient with malignant disease: Maternal–fetal conflict

D. FARINE AND E. N. KELLY

Introduction

One of the great tragedies of life is the situation faced by a pregnant woman confronted with the diagnosis of malignancy. On the one hand, she is full of hope and optimism with the thought of giving life, while at the same time faced with fear at the possibility of losing her own life while also possibly doing harm to her fetus. An exemplary case of maternal–fetal conflict arises when a pregnant woman is diagnosed to have a malignancy. The maternal interest is for an immediate treatment of the recently diagnosed tumor. Fetal well-being can be at times compromised by the presence of the tumor. However, the optimal therapy be it chemotherapy, radiotherapy or surgery almost always imposes much greater risks to the fetus than the malignancy *per se*. Therefore both the patient and her physician are often in a dilemma as to the optimal course.

Incidence

Pregnancy complicated by malignancy is unfortunately not uncommon. Pregnant women with cancer account for nearly 0.8% of all cancer cases in women. The American College of Obstetricians and Gynecologists estimates that about 3500 cases of cancer occur in pregnant women annually in the United States, or about 1 in 1000 pregnancies[1].

The incidence of specific cancers in pregnant women parallels that in women of childbearing age in general: cervical cancer is the most common, followed by breast cancer, melanoma and ovarian cancer.

Issues complicating the management of malignancy in the pregnant patient

The clinical decision on optimal treatment is extremely complicated for a variety of reasons.

1. Ethical and moral issues. The ethics regarding fetuses are still an evolving field and the relative importance of fetal well-being in comparison to maternal well-being differs between different ethicists, different religions and different cultures. The beliefs and moral stand could differ between the physicians and the family involved and at times even between the two parents.

2. The legal status of the fetus is not clear and its status differs in different legal jurisdictions. Although the fetus is not considered a person and thus does not consist of a legal entity and cannot sue the caregivers, the newborn (through his guardians) can sue for damages that occurred *in utero*. Furthermore, there have been several cases when the legal system has imposed a variety of therapies on the mother for the well-being of the fetus.

3. The effect of delayed therapy. In no other circumstances is there an often planned delay in the therapy of a patient with cancer. There is only limited information on the nature of the delays in therapy in patients with malignancies. These delays are usually related to delayed diagnosis, and the data published may be biased as clinicians may not be enthusiastic to report delays in therapy as these could be perceived as clinical failures. The data on malignancies in pregnancy are limited and anecdotal in nature since there are few large series analyzing different aspects of therapy. Randomized trials in this field are extremely difficult to undertake, and presently such rarely exist.

4. There is limited information on the effect of pregnancy on the biology of most tumors as well as the opposite, the effect of tumor on the pregnancy. These issues make any major clinical decisions extremely difficult. These decisions often include the following issues.

(a) Whether to terminate the pregnancy so that maternal therapy could be instituted immediately.

(b) Whether to institute chemotherapy, surgical, or radiation therapy without terminating the pregnancy. How does the pregnancy impact on the delivery of these therapies (e.g., surgical techniques, radiation, dosimetry, etc.) and their outcome? Should the therapy of choice be different in the presence of a pregnancy?

(c) What is the possible effect of therapy or avoidance of therapy on fetal well-being? Are there any long-term effects of the therapy on the fetus newborn child and eventually on the adult?

(d) How should the fetus be managed in terms of monitoring and therapy to enhance maturity.

(e) Who should provide medical and psychological support to the patient and her family and how (the oncologist, obstetrician/perinatologist, neonatologist, toxicologist, geneticist, psychologist) and what is the optimal set-up for such management?

(f) When is the optimal time for delivery, considering the risks of delaying therapy versus those of prematurity?

The purpose of this chapter is not to answer specific questions or to construct management schemes for specific tumors but to provide a framework for approaching some of these complex issues.

Ethical issues

The primary question in the context of possible fetal–maternal conflict pertains to the exact status of the fetus, or in other words: is the fetus a person? The answer to this question is not simple as can be evidenced by the schism between pro-life and pro-choice approaches when determining the balance between the value of fetal life and maternal autonomy. Different religions adopt different approaches to this issue, for example, in Judaism maternal interests precede fetal interest, while in Catholicism this relationship is more symmetrical. Some have suggested that the fetus becomes a person at some specific time in pregnancy. However, specific fetal anatomical or functional changes appear almost invariably to be a continuum. Therefore there is little agreement on any specific time in pregnancy when the fetus should be considered a person. Another approach is to consider the fetus to be a person once it could be viable outside the womb. However, once again there is a continuum in the chance of a specific fetus to survive. This probability is dependent on the gestational age at delivery, and the weight of the newborn as well on the expertise of the neonatologists taking care of the specific neonate and their set-up. The answer to these issues in our pluralistic society is to adopt some specific principles on which a practical ethical model can be developed. This model should accept and respect the diversity of approaches outlined above and, at the same time, be applicable to clinical medicine[2].

These two specific principles are as follows.

Respect for autonomy

The pregnant patient has a perspective on her best interests that are based on her values and beliefs. Therefore the patient should be in the position to have the freedom to choose alternatives based on these values and beliefs.

The fetus does not have a fully developed central nervous system and does not have beliefs or perspectives in his/her own interest. Therefore, there is no autonomy-based obligation of the physician to the fetus.

Beneficence

This requires the physician to assess objectively the various therapeutic options and to implement those which offer the patient the greatest balance of benefit over risks.

There is a beneficence obligation of the physician to the mother but also to the fetus.

Ethical conflicts

These two principles as applied to two persons, the mother and the fetus, may result in conflict. Such conflicts may include the following.

Conflict between maternal beneficence-based obligations of the physician and fetal beneficence-based obligations of the physician

The classic conflict in the constellation of pregnancy complicated by malignancy is between terminating the pregnancy for institution of maternal therapy or delaying maternal therapy for fetal maturity.

Conflict between fetal beneficence-based obligations of the mother and fetal beneficence-based obligations of the physician

Usually the mother and her physicians are in agreement as to the best interest of the fetus. However, the mother and the physician may differ on the need for specific treatment or investigation. This difference is not necessarily dependent on information given to the mother but may be due to different perception or acceptance of risks. For example, the physician may be reluctant to perform invasive tests (such as amniocentesis looking for the chromosomal effects of chemotherapy in the first trimester) if he believes that the risk is very low, while for the mother any such risk may be unacceptable.

Conflict between maternal autonomy-based obligations of the physician and fetal beneficence-based obligations of physician

These are more common conflicts. An example is a woman wishing to have a termination of pregnancy or very early cesarean section when the physician does not believe that the maternal risks of the disease are significant.

Conflict between maternal autonomy-based obligations of the physician and maternal beneficence-based obligations of physician

The classic example is blood administration to Jehovah witnesses. In cases of maternal malignancy, the patient may opt for a suboptimal therapy, experimental options or even nontraditional therapy, while the physician may evaluate this therapy to be nonbeneficial or even detrimental.

Legal aspects

The legal status of the fetus is complex. The fetus is not considered a person until delivery. Judgments such as Roe v. Wade established that the autonomy of women overrides any fetal rights. However, there are three different legal considerations that should be discussed in the context of a fetus that may be damaged as a consequence of cancer therapy in pregnancy.

1. A newborn (through his guardians) can sue for damages occurring *in utero* that could have been preventable. Furthermore, in one American precedent (Curlander v. Bio-science Laboratories) the court held that parents could be sued by their offspring if they allowed the baby to be born defective[3]. The implications of such a decision are that neither the parents nor the physicians may be immune from a legal suit by the damaged baby even if proper counselling was provided and informed decisions have been made.
2. A newborn may sue for wrongful life. The initial suits for wrongful life in the 1960s were in cases involving congenital rubella syndrome. The parents successfully claimed in these suits that they should have been informed of this specific outcome and offered a termination of pregnancy. Analysis of these suits suggests that, in the context of pregnancy complicated by malignancies, such cases are unlikely to be either pursued or to be successful if the parents are properly counselled.
3. Fetal rights. There have been a limited number of cases where courts forced procedures or therapy on women for fetal reasons. There were 21 such documented cases by 1987[4]. These included: 15 court orders for

cesarean delivery, 3 for detention in women with diabetes who refused treatment. There were two court orders for fetal intrauterine transfusions. Court orders were obtained in 86% of the 21 cases where they were sought. In the majority of these cases (88%) the order was granted within 6 hours of request. There was a criticism of the fact that, in 81% of cases, the women were Black, Hispanic or Asian and that 25% did not speak English as their primary language[5]. It should be also stressed that, in three of the first five cases of court-ordered cesarean sections, these women delivered vaginally without any complications casting major doubt on the ability of physicians to accurately predict outcome.

We are aware of only one case of court-ordered cesarean section in a woman with terminal cancer who was dying in an intensive care unit of a large bone tumor metastasis occupying her lung[6]. The initial plan was to perform a cesarean section at 28 weeks' gestation. However, at 26.5 weeks the hospital asked for a court decision for a cesarean section. The judge granted this motion in spite of the fact the woman's wishes were not clear and that her own physician did not want to perform the cesarean delivery. The baby died few hours after delivery and the mother died few days later. This decision was overturned three years later by a higher court that decided that the woman's wishes should have been followed in this case and these were not properly determined.[5]

The effects of pregnancy on tumor

There is usually no effect of the pregnancy *per se* on the rate of tumor growth or dissemination. There is often a delay in diagnosis of malignancies in pregnant women as symptoms are attributed to pregnancy, physical signs such as abdominal distention are masked by the pregnancy, and invasive tests are delayed. Therapy may be also delayed in a pregnant woman and these factors may compromise outcome. Some tumors have hormonal receptors (e.g., receptors for sex hormones) and at least theoretically these tumors may grow more rapidly in a milieu with increased hormonal levels. However, in tumors such as breast cancer there was no evidence of more aggressive biological behavior[7].

The effects of tumor on pregnancy

There have been only a few cases of maternal tumors crossing the placental barrier and extending to the fetus as outlined in the chapter on fetal tumors. However, advanced tumors have been associated with intrauterine growth

Table 2.1. *Neonatal survival by gestational age*

Reference (1)	23	24	25	26	27	28	29	30
Toronto–MSH 90–94 (8)	17%	53%	68%	87%	92%	93%	93%	98%
Toronto–WCH 88–91 (9)	5%	25%	70%	80%	90%	90%	96%	
Hopkins 88–91 (10)	17%	56%	80%					
NIHCD 89–90 (11)	15%	54%	59%	71%				
Connec 89–93 (12)	27%	56%	64%	87%				
Vancouver 83–89 (13)		16%	43%	55%	63%	87%		

MSH: Mount Sinai Hospital.   WCH: Women's College Hospital.

restrictions and stillbirths as outlined in several chapters of this book. Therefore, it is prudent to establish fetal monitoring to ensure fetal well-being even in the absence of active maternal therapy that could further jeopardize the fetus.

The optimal time of delivery

One of the major dilemmas in managing a woman with malignant disease is the timing of delivery. The physician needs to balance the risk to the health of the mother by postponement of chemotherapy and the risk to the fetus of either the initiation of therapy using potentially toxic chemicals or terminating the pregnancy.

The question is then, what is the optimal time? Traditionally, delivery at 34 weeks of gestation was considered safe with little risk of respiratory distress syndrome (RDS) or intraventricular hemorrhage (IVH). However, recent advances in perinatology and neonatology have shown significantly improved survival in lower gestational ages (see Table 2.1).

Survival at 27 weeks and beyond, as the Table shows, is 90% in the more recent studies and so one could recommend delivery at 30 weeks and possibly 28 weeks. Delivery in these cases should take place in a high-risk perinatal centre. The condition of the fetus must be optimized by attempting to mature the lungs using antenatal steroids ± thyrotropin releasing hormone (TRH) and/or other therapies should they become available and by the use of surfactant postnatally if required. In a recent report, Maher *et al*[14] showed that infants of women given betamethazone before delivery had a lower incidence of mortality/morbidity in comparison controls. RDS and IVH were significantly lower in the 29–31-week gestational age.

The next issue to be addressed is whether the quality of survival has improved, should one make the decision to deliver earlier. Here the information is less clear. Kitchen *et al* (1991)[15] comparing two epochs of babies 500–999 g demonstrated increased survival but no change in the percentage (%) of intact survival. Blaymore-Bier *et al* 1994[16] reporting on babies less than 750 grams over the period 1980–1990 similarly demonstrated improved survival but unchanging rate of handicap. Robertson *et al*[17], comparing two epochs 1978–79 and 1988–89 in babies 500 to 1250 g also demonstrated improving survival with no change in the percentage of handicapped survivors, although they noted that handicap rates were highest for those of lowest birth weights. Perlman 1995[18], again comparing two epochs 1980–84 and 1985–89, and in very low birth weight babies (< 800 g), noted a decreased incidence of handicap mainly due to a drop in incidence of blindness. In Robertson's study[17] the incidence of disability in the 1000–1250 g infants was 15% including 7% incidence of mental retardation. In the Scottish Low Birthweight Study[19] evaluating all infants born in Scotland in 1984 weighing less than 1750 g, overall 16% were disabled at 4.5 years, in the 1000–1499 g the incidence of moderate to severe disability was 15.4% and in the 1500 to 1740 g group it was 12.7%. This last study reported on a 1984 cohort, before the routine use of surfactant. Asztalos[9] in her study in the period 1988–90 ($n = 233$) with a 6.5% mortality, found a 78% intact survival in babies born at 28 to 29 weeks in those followed to two years ($n = 173$). Many studies have shown intraventricular hemorrhage to be one of the major predictors of outcome, both at two years and at school-age. From our own database (Table 2.2) one can see that the incidence of IVH decreases as gestational age and birth weight increase and that the incidence of major ultrasound abnormalities (IVH gr III and IV) and cysts (including periventricular leukomalacia) is approximately 5% in babies above 1250 g or at or above 30 weeks. Therefore it seems prudent to recommend delivery at a minimum of 30 weeks' gestation to allow preterm infants to be born with a low risk of major handicap and to permit initiation of maternal antineoplastic chemotherapy or radiation.

Summary: general guidelines for management

Team approach

In order to evaluate properly the risks involved and counsel the patient and a family, a team approach is required. The team should include the physicians involved in the management of the tumors (oncologists specializing in radiation and/or chemotherapy, surgeons and other relevant specialties), obstetrician or perinatologist and pediatrician or preferably a neonatologist. Nurses from the above disciplines are essential to develop a management

Table 2.2. *MSH NICU 1990–1994 Stats*

By birth weight:

Birth weight	<750	751–1000	1001–1250	1251–1500	= >1501	Total
Admissions	203	342	331	384	2641	3901
Died	91	40	13	9	48	201
Normal HUS	53(%)	174	205	175	300	907
IVH I	18	46	40	46	29	179
IVH II	19	29	15	6	7	76
IVH III	11	16	14	7	3	51
IVH IV	17	19	5	1	4	46
Cysts	9	14	24	12	22	81

By gestational age:

Gest. age (wk)	= 28	= 29	= 30	= 31	= 32	> 32	Total
Admissions	177	192	227	293	339	2178	3406
Died	12	15	5	7	6	32	77
Normal HUS	110	99	119	131	92	171	722
IVH I	20	23	19	31	17	9	119
IVH II	7	6	7	4	1	4	29
IVH III	5	7	2	2	2	1	19
IVH IV	1	3	1	1	0	3	9
Cysts	9	7	6	10	4	17	53

HUS: Head ultrasound.
IVH: Intraventricular hemorrhage.
MSH: Mount Sinai Hospital, Toronto.

plan and in implementing it. The team members have to educate one another on the issues relevant to the case from their own disciplines. Only such a team can provide proper counselling and offer optimal management of the mother and her unborn baby. Although such teams could be created *de novo* for specific cases, it is conceivable that an ongoing team is more efficient in the interdisciplinary discussions and management plan development. To this core team other health professionals such as clinical pharmacologists, radiologists, etc. involved in the care of a specific patient can be added as required. An involvement of an ethicist and/or the hospital lawyers may be required in unusual cases.

The team should discuss freely all the relevant issues with the patient, trying to develop a plan for the management of the pregnancy. The wishes of the patient should guide the team after proper counselling has taken place.

The set-up

It is important to provide care by the same team throughout pregnancy. This allows the creation of trust, ongoing counselling and ensures that the wishes of the patient are respected throughout her pregnancy. The management of such cases should take place in a tertiary centre that can provide care for complicated pregnancies, very premature neonates and optimal oncology care.

Psychological support

There should be special attention to the psychological needs of the patient and her family. Although oncologists, surgeons, perinatologists and neonatologists are quite aware of the psychological aspects of their own disciplines, they are less versed in these issues as applied to the other disciplines. Active involvement of the nursing staff and social workers from these disciplines may provide the backbone of psychological support. Involvement of either psychologists or psychiatrists may often be required.

Fetal monitoring

The fetus should be properly monitored (see chapter on fetal monitoring) as often these fetuses are growth restricted and at higher risks of intrauterine death. Maternal reassurance of fetal well-being is of paramount importance for relieving maternal anxiety and concerns.

Fetal therapy for prevention of neonatal complications

Maternal administration of corticosteroids reduces the risks of neonatal respiratory distress syndrome (RDS) as well as the risks of neonatal intraventricular hemorrhage (IVH). Such therapy should be offered at 24–34 weeks of gestation if there is a possibility that preterm delivery or early delivery may be indicated[14].

Optimal time of delivery

This should be individually assessed based on the risk of delaying therapy versus the risks of prematurity. The mortality rate after 30 weeks of gestation has been shown to be invariably low in tertiary centres and rarely exceeds 1%. Therefore the "classic optimal time to delivery" suggested in the past in major textbooks to be 34 weeks gestation[20] or when lung maturity is confirmed[21], should be re-examined and probably moved to an earlier time when needed.

References

1. Waalen J: Pregnancy poses tough questions for cancer treatment. *J Natl Cancer Inst* 1991; 83: 900–1.
2. Chervenak FA, McCullough LB: Perinatal ethics: a practical method of analysis of obligations to mother and fetus. *Obstet Gynecol* 1985; 66: 442–6.
3. Engelhardt T: Current controversies in obstetrics: wrongful life and forced fetal surgical procedures. *Am J Obstet Gynecol* 1985; 151: 313–18.
4. Kolder VEB, Gallagher JD, Parsons MT: Court ordered obstetrical interventions. *New Engl J Med* 1987; 316: 1192–6.
5. Curran WJC: Court ordered cesarean sections receive judicial defeat. *Law Med Notes* 1990; 323: 489–92.
6. Tuohey JF: Terminal care and the pregnant woman; ethical reflections on in re: A.C. *Pediatrics* 1991; 88: 1268–73.
7. Baron RH: Dispelling the myths of pregnancy-associated breast cancer. *Oncol Nurs Forum* 1994; 21(3): 507–12.
8. Mount Sinai Hospital Database 1990–94 (MSH unpublished).
9. Asztalos EV, Zayack MD, Shennan AT: Is there room for optimism? Two year outcome in premature infants born under 30 weeks' gestation in a regional perinatal centre (1988–91). *Pediatr Res* 1995; 35: 213A.
10. Allen MC, Donohue PK, Dusman AE: The limit of viability – neonatal outcome if infants born at 22 to 25 weeks' gestation. *New Engl J Med* 1993; 329: 1597–601.
11. Hack M, Wright LL, Shankaran S, Tyson JE, Horbar JD, Bauer CR, Younes N: Very low birth weight outcomes of the National Institute of Child Health and Human Development Neonatal Network. *Am J Obstet Gynecol* Nov. 1989 to Oct. 1990.
12. Hussain N, Galal M, Ehrenkranz RA, Herson VC, Rowe JC: Mortality and morbidity of the 22 to 27 weeks' gestational age infants born at high risk perinatal units in Connecticut in the surfactant era. *Pediatr Res* 1994; 35: 274A.
13. Synnes AR, Ling EWY, Whitfield MF, MacKinnon M, Lopes L, Wong G, Effer SB: Perinatal outcomes of a large cohort of extremely low gestational age infants (23 to 28 completed weeks of gestation). *J. Pediatr* 1994; 125: 952–60.
14. Maher JE, Cliver SP, Goldenberg RL, Davis RO, Copper RL and The March of Dimes Multicenter Study Group: The effect of corticosteroid therapy in the very premature infant. *Am J Obstet Gynecol* 1994; 170: 869–73.
15. Kitchen WH, Doyle LW, Ford GW, Murton LJ, Keith CG, Rickards AL, Kelly E, Callanan C: Changing outcome of infants weighing 500 to 999 grams at birth: a hospital study. *J Pediatr* 1991; 118: 938–43.
16. Blaymore-Bier J, Pezzullo J, Kim E, Oh W, Garcia-Coll C, Vohr BR: Outcome of extremely low-birth weight infants. *Acta Paediatr* 1994; 83: 1244–8.
17. Robertson CMT, Hrynchyshyn GJ, Etches PC, Pain KS: Population-based study of the incidence, complexity, and severity of neurologic disability among survivors weighing 500 through 1250 grams at birth. *Pediatrics* 1992; 90: 750–5.
18. Perlman M, Claris O, Hao Y, Pandit P, Whyte H, Chipman M, Liu M: Secular changes in the outcomes to eighteen to twenty-four months of age of extremely low birth weight infants, with adjustment for changes in risk factors and severity of illness. *J Pediatr* 1995; 126: 75–87.

19. The Scottish Low Birthweight Study Group: I. Survival, growth, neuromotor and sensory impairment. *Arch Dis Child* 1992; 67: 675–81.
20. Creasy RK, Resnik R (eds.): *Maternal–Fetal Medicine*. 1994 p. 1115, WB Saunders Co. Philadelphia, London, Toronto, Montreal, Sydney, Tokyo.
21. Cunningham FG, MacDonald PC, Gant NF, Leveno KJ, Gilstrap LC (eds.): *Williams Obstetrics* 1993, p. 1274, Appleton & Lange, Norwalk, Connecticut.

3

Changes in drug disposition during pregnancy and their clinical implications

G. KOREN

For obvious reasons, almost none of the research projects involved in understanding pregnancy-induced changes in drug disposition has been conducted in women with cancer or in other women receiving cancer chemotherapy for adverse indications.

This chapter, therefore, will overview general principles governing changes in drug disposition during pregnancy, assuming that these mechanisms will be operative for cancer drugs too.

Clinical case

One of your patients, a G1 P0 epileptic woman (65 kg in late gestation) who was maintained on 400 mg/d of phenytoin taken in two equal doses every 12 hours has just had her first and only grand mal seizure during pregnancy at 26 weeks of gestation. Upon arrival to the emergency room her phenytoin level was 5 mg/L 10 hours after her evening dose. Three trough levels taken before, at various times during pregnancy, were between 12 and 17 mg/L. What are your thoughts about the mechanism leading to this seizure?

Introduction

While the potential hazards to the unborn baby from medications administered to the pregnant woman are a major concern, one should be very careful not to neglect the maternal part of the fetomaternal unit. It has been universally agreed that the well-being of the mother should dictate her need for drug therapy and that one should not subject pregnant women to suboptimal therapy that may endanger them.

Pregnancy is associated with a plethora of physiological changes that may affect the natural course of diseases, the way the body handles drugs, or both. This chapter summarizes major changes in the pharmacokinetics of drugs in pregnancy and their clinical implications. Whereas Chapters 17 and 18 deal with the effects of maternal diseases on the reproductive outcome, this chapter focuses on the possible need for alterations in drug therapy in pregnancy to deal with pharmacokinetic and pathophysiological changes.

Pharmacokinetics of the maternal–fetal unit

Several pharmacokinetic models have been used to describe the movement of different drugs between the maternal and fetal circulations[1]. In general, two principal groups of changes characterize pregnancy with respect to drug disposition.

Alterations in drug kinetics due to maternal changes

There is a gradual increase in renal function in pregnancy. This will result in an augmented elimination rate of agents that are excreted by the kidney (e.g., ampicillin, gentamicin, amikacin, digoxin)[2–5]. Distribution volume may be altered during pregnancy because of increases to 50% in blood (plasma) volume and 30% in cardiac output[6–8]. A parallel 50% increment in renal flow and a substantial increase of uterine blood flow to 600–700 mL/min also take place. During pregnancy there is a mean increase of 8 L in body water: 60% of it is distributed to the placenta, fetus, and amniotic fluid, and 40% is distributed to maternal tissues[6,9–12]. Consequently, a decrease in the serum concentrations of many drugs has been documented. It is very likely that lower serum concentrations in pregnancy will be noted, especially with drugs having a relatively small distribution volume which corresponds to water compartments.

Of potential clinical importance, the protein binding of several antiepileptic drugs including phenytoin, diazepam, and valproic acid has been shown to decrease significantly toward the last trimester of pregnancy[13]. These drugs are discussed later in this chapter.

Changes in hepatic elimination patterns during pregnancy are less consistent. Hepatic blood flow appears to be unchanged during pregnancy[1]. However, there is evidence that the elimination rate of clindamycin, which is metabolized by the liver, is increased during pregnancy[3], suggesting a possible increase in hepatic clearance. It is possible that the faster elimination of trimethoprim/sulfamethoxazole observed during pregnancy is due to higher liver clearance, although increased renal clearance may be the major determinant of this change[14].

Table 3.1. *Selected drugs having lower serum concentrations during pregnancy and relevant pharmacokinetic changes* [3,4,13, 15–21]

Drug	Elimination halt-time	Vd	Clearance	Protein binding
Amikacin	↓			
Ampicillin	↓	↑	↑	↓
Cephalosporins	↓	↓		
Erythromycin				
Gentamicin	→			
Kanamycin	→			
Methicillin	↑			
Nitrofurantoin				
Oxacillin		↑	↑	
Phenobarbitol			↑	↓
Phenytoin		↑	↑	↓

Vd: Volume of distribution.

The decrease in drug–protein binding discussed previously may also account for higher clearance rates of drugs in pregnancy, as it is the free fraction which is accessible to the metabolizing systems. Studies in epileptic women have shown an increase in the clearance of phenytoin during pregnancy, accounting for lower serum concentrations[12].

As shown in Table 3.1, the above-mentioned changes in the pharmacokinetics of many drugs administered during pregnancy result in a decrease in serum concentrations when compared to levels measured in nonpregnant women. Thus, the standard dose schedule may result in lower concentrations in pregnancy and, as discussed later, these changes may have important implications in treating the pregnant woman.

The effects of the placental–fetal compartment

Almost all drugs have been shown to cross the placenta and to appear in measurable concentrations in the fetal blood. Several determinants govern the movement of drugs across the placental barrier and determine the materno-fetal ratio of concentrations. In general, the ratio between drug concentration in the fetus versus the mother is different from (in most cases less than) unity (Table 3.2).

Differences in protein binding

Fetal protein appears to bind less avidly various drugs, including ampicillin and benzylpenicillin[33]. Conversely, no differences between maternal and

Table 3.2. *Fetomaternal concentration ratio of antibiotics* [3,22–32]

Drug	Fetomaternal ratio
Ampicillin	0.38–0.87
Cephalosporins	0.13–1.0
Clindamycin	0.4–0.5
Dicloxacillin	0.07–0.27
Gentamicin	0.21–1.0
Methicillin	0.83–1.43
Penicillin G	0.06–0.7

fetal protein binding were found for methicillin and dicloxacillin[30]. Salicylates, on the other hand, appear to have a more extensive binding to fetal than to maternal protein[34].

During pregnancy there is a gradual decrease in the concentrations of maternal albumin and an increase in the concentrations of fetal albumin. Consequently, at different times during pregnancy, different fetal/maternal ratios of albumin occur. At term, it appears that fetal albumin concentrations are equal or even higher than in the mother. The degree of protein binding of a drug is an important determinant of its movement across the placenta. The least protein-bound drugs (e.g., digoxin, ampicillin, 20%) reach higher concentrations in the fetus and in the amniotic fluid. Drugs with high protein binding (e.g., dicloxacillin, 96%) achieve higher maternal and lower fetal concentrations because only the free fraction of the drug crosses the placental barrier. Since, however, additional determinants other than protein binding may play an important role in placental passage, drugs such as sulfisoxazole reach therapeutic concentrations in the fetus in spite of their high protein binding.

Differences in pH

Fetal blood pH is slightly lower than the maternal. The pH gradient may influence the movement of drugs according to their pK_a. This results in an apparent fall in fetal concentrations of nonionized drugs and leads to a concentration gradient, leading to net movement from maternal to fetal systems[35]. This mechanism is commonly referred to as "ion trapping." In contrast to weak bases, ion trapping induced from fetal to maternal circulations is likely to occur with weak acids.

Other effects

Other important determinants of drug transport across the placenta are water/lipid solubility, molecular weight, and the surface available for diffusion. A good example of the different effects on placental passage is the higher concentration of trimethoprim in the fetus than in the mother, corresponding to its relatively low protein binding (42–46%), pK_a of 6.6, and poor water solubility. Sulfamethoxazole, on the other hand, has good water solubility at physiological pH and therefore has more difficulties in crossing the lipid–placental barrier. Both drugs appear to reach the amniotic fluid, and their concentration ratio there corresponds closely to that in the fetal serum[36].

Following repeated doses of drugs, concentrations measured in the fetus appear to be higher than following a single dose[37,38]. Repeated high bolus injections of ampicillin or gentamicin yield higher concentrations in fetal serum and amniotic fluid than after a single bolus, and after a single intravenous dose a peak umbilical concentration is achieved within 30–60 min.

Fetoplacental drug elimination

Drug metabolism has been documented by the fetal liver as early as 7–8 weeks of pregnancy. Virtually all enzymatic processes, including phase 1 (oxidation, dehydrogenation, reduction, hydrolysis, etc.) and phase 2 (glucuronidation, methylation, acetylation, etc.) have been documented in the fetal liver[39]. However, the degree of activity is very low in most cases when compared to the adult liver. Similarly, drug-metabolizing activity has been demonstrated in human placental tissue. In summary, the placentofetal unit contributes only marginally to the total elimination capacity of drugs by the maternal body. As pregnancy progresses, higher amounts of antimicrobials are excreted into the amniotic fluids through fetal urine. This process depends upon maturation of the fetal kidney.

In general, metabolites are more polar than their parent compounds and are therefore less likely to cross the placental barrier. As a result, metabolites may accumulate in various tissues of the fetus or may be recovered from the amniotic fluid. It has been shown that thiamphenicol achieves higher concentrations in the umbilical vein than in the umbilical artery, reflecting some degree of extraction of the drug by the fetus, probably by renal excretion[32].

Clinical implications

As reflected in the preceding discussion, a variety of drugs appear to achieve lower serum concentrations during pregnancy. For agents that exhibit good correlation between serum concentrations and pharmacological effects, this may mean that, during pregnancy, patients may be at a higher risk of suboptimal therapy.

Anticonvulsants

As discussed above, there is good evidence that the serum concentrations of phenytoin, phenobarbital[40], ethosuximide[41], and carbamazepine[42] decrease as pregnancy progresses. Some authors observed an increase in the frequency of seizures as phenytoin clearance increased in pregnancy and plasma levels fell[40]. A variety of reasons have been put forward to explain this fall in drug concentrations in pregnancy.

1. Increase in extracellular fluid and tissue volume, leading to increase in distribution volume of the drug.
2. Decreased plasma–protein binding, leading to more free drug available for biotransformation. It should be mentioned, however, that higher free drug concentration may secure antiepileptic effect even in the presence of lower total drug level, as it is the free drug that reaches the brain.
3. Folate supplementation, given to the pregnant woman, may increase liver metabolism of phenytoin[41].
4. Increase in glomerular filtration rate (GFR), leading to faster clearance rates of drugs eliminated by the kidney.

The question of whether epilepsy is worsened during pregnancy is of extreme importance; current evidence, however, is inconclusive: Schmidt reviewed 2162 pregnancies and could not detect a clear pattern, as some 23% reported improvement, 53% no change, and 24% worsened[43]. Yet, other studies suggest that epilepsy with at least one seizure per month is likely to worsen in pregnancy[44].

Changes in seizure frequency in pregnancy may stem from fluid and sodium retention, hyperventilation, a rise in estrogen levels, emotional and psychological problems, and the tendency of drug levels to fall[13]. Although presently no research has addressed the contribution of each factor, there are well-documented cases to prove the importance of adequate serum concentrations during pregnancy[13,41].

Caring for the pregnant epileptic patient must therefore incorporate careful monitoring of serum concentrations and appropriate adjustment of the antiepileptic dose. After pregnancy, most women will need lower dosages, and failure to adjust their schedule may lead to drug toxicity.

Lithium

The antidepressant lithium is eliminated almost entirely by the kidney. The pregnancy-induced increase in the GFR is consistent therefore with lower serum concentration so lithium was reported sporadically during pregnancy[45]. Because, in many cases, lithium exerts its pharmacological effects at nearly toxic levels, the drop in serum concentrations may lead to suboptimal therapy.

After giving birth, with the return of the GFR to its prepregnancy values, patients may need reduction of their doses.

Some lithium is reabsorbed by the renal tubule, and this process is in competition with sodium reabsorption. Pregnant patients with toxemia are kept on a restricted sodium intake, and therefore they may experience higher levels of lithium owing to higher renal reabsorption of the cation.

Digoxin

Similar to lithium, digoxin is eliminated in humans mainly by renal excretion and therefore is expected to maintain lower steady-state concentrations in pregnancy. When measured at term, digoxin serum concentrations were found in five pregnant women to be almost twofold lower than one month later[5].

Ampicillin

Since ampicillin is one of the most widely used antibiotics, knowledge of its pharmacokinetics in pregnancy may yield valuable information about the dose requirement during gestation. Philipson, who studied the disposition of ampicillin once during and again after pregnancy, found the plasma concentration to be 50% lower during gestation owing to both the larger distribution volume and faster clearance rate[2]. Similar to digoxin and lithium, ampicillin is eliminated mainly through the kidney, and the twofold decrease in its levels is consistent with that described for digoxin.

Other drugs

Similar observations have been documented with cephalosporins, clindamycin, erythromycin, kanamycin, amikacin, tobramycin, nitrofurantoin,

Table 3.3. *Therapeutic serum concentrations of drugs commonly monitored in clinical practice, and documented changes in pregnancy*

| Drug | Units of therapeutic concentration | | Documented changes in drug concentration during pregnancy |
	Metric	SI	
Amikacin	Peak < 20–30 µg/mL		↓
	Trough < 5–10 µg/mL		
Amiodarone	< 2.5 µg/mL		
Carbamazepine	4–12 µg/mL	17–51 µM	↓
Chloramphenicol	< 25 µg/mL		
Cyclosporin	< 200–250 ng/mL		
Digoxin	0.5–2 ng/mL	0.7–2.6 nM	↓
Disopyramide	3–5 µg/mL	9–15	
Ethosximide	40–100 µg/mL	285–710 µM	↓
Gentamicin	Trough < 2–3 µg/mL		↓
	Peak < 8–10 µg/mL		
Lidocaine	1.5–5.0 µg/mL	6–21 µM	
Lithium		0.8–1.0 mM	↓
Methotrexate		< 5 µM 24 h after high dose	
Phenobarbitol	15–40 µg/mL	65–172 µM	↓
Phenytoin	10–20 µg/mL	39–79 µM	↓
Primidone	5–12 µg/mL	23–55 µM	
Procainamide	4–10 µg/mL	15–37 µM	
Quinidine	2.3–5.0 µg/mL	7–15 µM	
Theophylline	10–20 µg/mL	55–110 µM	
Tobramycin	Trough < 2–3 µg/mL		
	Peak < 8–10 µg/mL		
Valproic acid	50–100 µg/mL	347–693 µM	
Vancomycin	Trough < 10 µg/mL		
	Peak < 45 µg/mL		

and sulfamethoxazole trimethoprim[37]. In all instances, the lower serum concentrations during pregnancy could be attributed to pharmacokinetic changes.

Summary

It is conceivable that, for many drugs not yet studied, the same pattern of higher clearance rates and, therefore, lower steady-state concentrations prevails in pregnancy.

Drugs for which levels are monitored routinely are summarized in Table 3.3, along with their therapeutic range of serum concentrations. In monitoring chronic drug therapy in pregnancy, it is important to repeat measurements more often than routinely, since toward the end of pregnancy the physiological changes leading to lower serum concentrations are at their maximum. Decisions concerning increases of daily doses should incorporate the clinical status and the course of the disease, and they are best performed by the physician familiar with the woman's condition. It is important to remember not to "treat numbers;" while some patients have good control of their illness with low serum concentrations, others do not achieve favorable effects even at supratherapeutic drug levels. Concentrations of most drugs are not measured routinely in clinical practice; the general pattern delineated above should be borne in mind, since a higher clearance rate would mean that some pregnant women may need higher doses, especially if the regular (prepregnancy) schedule fails to produce the expected effects.

Answer

Epileptic women tend to have more seizures during pregnancy. After ruling out preeclampsia–eclampsia, electrolyte changes, and hypoalbuminemia, you should consider increased clearance rate of phenytoin as a cause for lower levels and the resulting seizures. To that end, you need to rule out decrease in compliance (i.e., the patient had not been taking her medications as before).

References

1. Krauer B, Krauer F: Drug kinetics in pregnancy. In *Handbook of Clinical Pharmacokinetics* (Gibaldi M, Prescott L, ed.), 1983, pp. 1–17, Section II, ADIS, New York.
2. Philipson A: Pharmacokinetics of ampicillin during pregnancy. *J Infect Dis* 1977; 136: 370–6.
3. Weinsten AJ, Gibbs RS, Gallagher M: Placental transfer of clindamycin and gentamicin in term pregnancy. *Am J Obstet Gynecol* 1976; 124: 688–91.
4. Bernard B, Abate M, Thielen PF, Attar H, Ballard CA, Wehnle PF: Maternal fetal pharmacological activity of amikacin. *J Infect Dis* 1977; 135: 925–32.
5. Roger ME, Willerson JT, Goldblatt A *et al*: Serum digoxin concentrations in the human fetus, neonate and infant. *New Engl J Med* 1972; 287: 1010–13.
6. Hytten FE, Leitch T. *The Physiology of Pregnancy*. 1971, Blackwell Oxford.
7. Pizani BBK, Campbell DM, McGillivray T: Plasma volume in normal pregnancy. *J Obstet Gynecol* 1973; 80: 884–7.
8. Walters WAW, Lengling Y: Blood volume and haemodynamics in pregnancy. In *Obstetrics and Gynecology*, Vol 2. 1975, pp. 301–302; Saunders, London.
9. Davidson JM, Hytten FE: Glomerular filtration during and after pregnancy. *J Obstet Gynecol* 1974; 81: 588–95.
10. Young IM: The placenta: blood flow and transfer. In *Modern Trends in Physiology*, pp. 214–244, Butterworth, London, 1972.

11. Kerr MG: Cardiovascular dynamics in pregnancy and labour. *Br Med Bull* 1968; 24: 19–24.
12. Rebound P, Groulade J, Groslambert P, Colomb M: The influence of normal pregnancy and the postpartum state on plasma proteins and lipids. *Am J Obstet Gynecol* 1963; 86: 820–8.
13. Perucca E, Richens A: Antiepileptic drugs, pregnancy and the newborn. In *Clinical Pharmacology in Obstetrics* (Lewis P, ed.), 1983, pp. 264–87, Wright PSG, Bristol, England.
14. Ylikorkala O, Sjostedt E, Jarvinen PA, Tikkanen R, Raines T: Trimethoprimsulfonamide combination administered orally and intravaginally in the first trimester of pregnancy: its absorption into serum and transfer to amniotic fluid. *Acta Obstet Gynecol Scand* 1973; 52: 229–234.
15. Bray RE, Boe RW, Johnson WL: Transfer of ampicillin into fetus and amniotic fluid from maternal plasma in late pregnancy. *Am J Obstet Gynecol* 1966; 96: 938–42.
16. Bernard B, Barton L, Abate M, Ballard CA: Maternal fetal transfer of cefazolin in the first twenty weeks of pregnancy. *J Infect Dis* 1977; 136: 377–82.
17. Philipson A, Saboth LD, Charles D: Erythromycin and clindamycin absorption and elimination in pregnant women. *Clin Pharmacol Ther* 1976; 19; 68–77.
18. Good RG, Johnson G: The placental transfer of kanamycin in late pregnancy. *Obstet Gynecol* 1971; 38: 60–2.
19. MacAuley MA, Berg SR, Charles D: Placental transfer of methicillin. *Am J Obstet Gynecol* 1973; 115: 58–65.
20. Amon K, Amon I, Huller H: Verteilung und Kinetik von Nitrofurantoin in der Fruhschwangerschaft. *Int J Clin Pharmacol Ther Toxicol* 1972; 63: 218–22.
21. Bastert G, Muller WG, Wallhauser KH, Hebauf H: Pharmacolinetishe Untersuchungen zum Ubertriff von Antibiotika in das Fruchtwasser am Enter der Schwangerschaft. 3. Oxacillin. *Geburtschilfe Perinatol* 1975; 179; 346–55.
22. Hirsch HA, Dreher E, Perrochet A, Schmid E: Transfer of ampicillin to the fetus and amniotic fluid during continuous infusion (steady state) and by repeated single intravenous injections to the mother. *Infection* 1974; 2: 207–12.
23. Croft I, Forster TC: Materno-fetal cephadine transfer in pregnancy. *Antimicrob Agents Chemother* 1978; 14: 924–6.
24. Barr W, Graham RM: Placental transmission of cephaloxidine. *J Obstet Gynecol* 1947; 74: 739–45.
25. Hirsch HA, Herbet S, Lang R, Dettli L, Goblinger A: Transfer of a new cephalosporin antibiotic to the fetus and the amniotic fluid during a continuous infusion (steady state) and single repeated intravenous injections to the mother. *Anz Fonsch* 1974; 24: 1474–8.
26. MacAuley MA, Abou-Sabe M, Charles D: Placental transfer of dicloxacillin at term. *Am J Obstet Gynecol* 1968; 102: 1162–8.
27. Forreres L, Paz M, Martin G, Gobernado M: New studies on placental transfer of fosfomycin. *Chemotherapy* 1977 (suppl 1): 175–9.
28. Daubenfeld O, Modde H, Hirsch HA: Transfer of gentamicin to the foetus and amniotic fluid during a steady state in the mother. *Arch Gynecol* 1974; 217: 233–40.
29. Yoshioka H, Monma T, Matsudo S: Placental transfer of gentamicin. *J Pediatr* 1972; 80: 121–3.
30. Depp R, Kind AC, Kirby, WMM, Johnson WL: Transplacental passage of

methicillin and dicloxacillin into the fetus and amniotic fluid. *Am J Obstet Gynecol* 1970; 107: 1054–7.

31. Charles D: Placental transmission of antibiotics. *J Obstet Gynecol* 1954; 61: 790–7.
32. Plomp TA, Moes RAA, Thiery M: Placental transfer of thiamphenicol in term pregnancy. *Fur J Obstet Gynecol Reprod Biol* 1977; 7: 383–8.
33. Tucker GT, Boyes RN, Bridenbaugh PO: Binding of anilide-type local anesthetics in human plasma. II. Implications *in vivo*, with special reference to transplacental distribution. *Anesthesiology* 1970; 33: 304–14.
34. Levy G: Salicylate pharmacokinetics in the human neonate. In *Basic and Therapeutic Aspects of Perinatal Pharmacology* (Morselli P, Garattini C, Sereni Y, eds.), 1975, pp. 319–330; Raven Press, New York.
35. Asling JH, Way EL: Placental transfer of drugs. In *Fundamentals of Drug Metabolism and Drug Disposition* (La Du, Mandel, Way Y, eds.), 1972, p. 88; Williams & Wilkins, Baltimore.
36. Walter AM, Heilmeyer L: *Antibiotika-Fibel*, Vol 4. Auflage. Thieme, Stuttgart, 1975.
37. Philipson A: Pharmacokinetics of antibiotics in pregnancy and labour. *Clin Pharmacokinet* 1979; 4: 297–309.
38. Chow AW, Jewesson PJ: Pharmacokinetics and safety of antimicrobial agents during pregnancy. *Rev Infect Dis* 1985; 7: 287–313.
39. Juchau MR, Chao ST, Omiecinski CJ: Drug metabolism by the human fetus. In *Handbook of Clinical Pharmacokinetics* (Gibaldi M, Prescott L, eds.), 1983, pp. 58–78; Section II, ADIS, New York.
40. Dam M, Mygind KJ, Christiansen J: Antiepileptic drugs: plasma clearance during pregnancy. *Epileptology* 1976; Jan. 3: 179–83.
41. Eadie MJ, Lander CM, Tyrer JH: Plasma drug level monitoring in pregnancy. In *Handbook of Clinical Pharmacokinetics* (Gibaldi M, Prescott L, eds), 1983, pp. 53–62, Section IV, ADIS, NY.
42. Dam M, Christiansen J, Munck O, Mygind KI: Antiepileptic drugs: metabolism in pregnancy. *Clin Pharmacokinet* 1979; 4: 53–62.
43. Schmidt D: The effect of pregnancy on the natural history of epilepsy. In *Epilepsy, Pregnancy and the Child* (Janz D, Bossi L, Dam M, ed.), 1981, pp. 3–14; Raven Press, New York.
44. Knight AH, Rhind EG: Epilepsy and pregnancy: a study of 153 pregnancies in 59 patients. *Epilepsia* 1975; 16: 99–110.
45. Schou M, Amidsen A, Steenstrup DR: Lithium and pregnancy. II: hazards to women given lithium during pregnancy and delivery. *Br Med J* 1973; 2: 137–8.

4

The role of the placenta in the biotransformation of carcinogenic compounds

L. DEREWLANY AND G. KOREN

Introduction

In this chapter we shall discuss the metabolic role of the placenta in activating or deactivating molecules which may be carcinogenic. We have recently described the metabolism of two primary arylamine substrates by acetyl coenzyme A-dependent arylamine N-acetyltransferase (NAT) in human placenta[1,2]. Another group of substrates for the NAT enzyme are the carcinogenic arylamines such as benzidine, β-naphthylamine and 4-aminobiphenyl. These compounds are generated industrially in the manufacture of dyestuffs, pesticides and plastics. In addition, these chemical entities may be found in the environment as products of fuel combustion and in cigarette smoke at concentrations for which there is evidence of carcinogenicity in human (1 to 22 ng per cigarette in mainstream smoke)[1]. Highly mutagenic aromatic amines have also been identified in protein-containing foods as products of the cooking process[2,3]. These are of particular toxicologic interest since up to 35% of cancer deaths are believed to be linked to diet[4].

The association between cancer and exposure to aromatic amines was first identified in the late 1800s when cancer of the urinary bladder was linked to exposure to compounds used in the manufacture of aniline dyes[5]. However, the first link between an individual aromatic amine entity and cancer was not made until 1938 when β-naphthylamine was shown to induce urinary bladder cancer in dogs[6]. Epidemiologic studies have now definitely linked three aromatic amine compounds (benzidine, β-naphthylamine, 4-aminobiphenyl) to cancer in humans[7]. Other aromatic amine compounds have been shown to be carcinogenic in laboratory animals and are thus suspected to be carcinogenic in humans as well.

Many mutagenic and carcinogenic compounds are known to exert their toxic effects only after metabolic activation to reactive electrophiles which

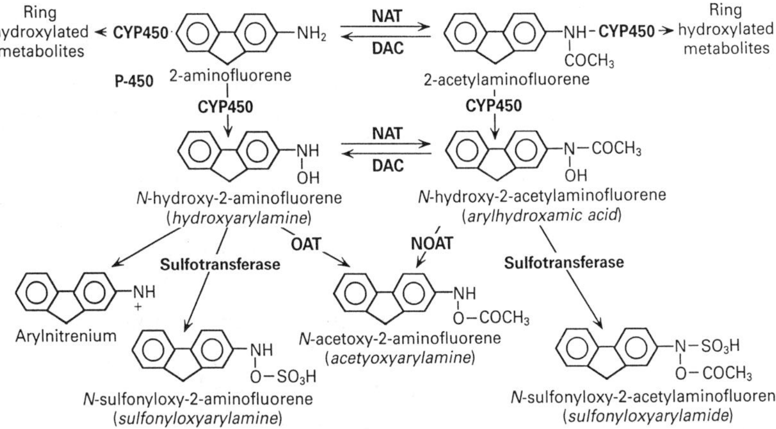

Fig. 4.1 Metabolic activation pathways of 2-aminofluorene and 2-acetylamino-fluorene. Enzymes involved are: cytochromes P-450 (CYP450); *N*-acetyltransferase (NAT); arylhydroxamic acid *N*,O-acyltransferase (NOAT); *N*-hydroxyarylamine O-acetyltransferase (OAT); deacetylase (DAC);sulfotransferase.

covalently bind to critical cell targets[8]. This is the mechanism of action attributed to the carcinogenic arylamines. The metabolism of a prototype carcinogenic arylamine, 2-aminofluorene (AF) is shown in Fig. 4.1. 2-aminofluorene is a synthetic arylamine compound, and its metabolism has been extensively studied in the laboratory.

Chemically reactive electrophiles formed from 2-aminofluorene and 2-acetylaminofluorene which can react with nucleophilic sites include the acetoxyarylamine, sulfonyloxyarylamine, sulfonyloxyarylamide and aryl-nitrenium ion shown in Fig. 4.1. *In vivo*, the macromolecular nucleophilic targets for these compounds are DNA, RNA and protein. The covalent binding of reactive electrophiles to critical cell targets may ultimately (if not repaired by intracellular repair mechanisms) result in carcinogenesis, mutagenesis, cytotoxicity and genotoxicity. These compounds have also been shown to be teratogenic, as will be discussed below.

The initial step in the metabolic process is *N*-hydroxylation to form hydroxamic acids. This reaction is mediated by the cytochrome P450 monooxygenases[9]. Ring hydroxylation of the arylamines to epoxide or phenolic compounds by monooxygenase or peroxidase enzymes is not thought to be an important activation pathway[10]. Although the hydroxamic acid metabolites will form DNA adducts when administered *in vivo*, these compounds undergo further activation to form more toxic, ultimate carcinogens.

The reactive sulfate ester metabolites (sulfonyloxyarylamine and sulfonyloxyarylamide) are formed via the action of sulfotransferase. The highly reactive acetoxyarylamine compounds is formed by the actions of acetyl coenzyme A-dependent arylamine *N*-acetyltransferase (NAT), acetyl coenzyme A-dependent *N*-hydroxyarylamine (NAT), acetyl coenzyme A-dependent *N*-hydroxyarylamine *O*-acetyltransferase (OAT), arylhydroxamic acid *N*, *O*-acyltransferase (NOAT) and deacetylase (DAC). Fig. 4.1 shows the metabolic pathways involved in the formation of reactive metabolites from AF and/or 2-acetylaminofluorene (AAF) by these enzymes. However, it is important to remember that the actual metabolite formed *in vivo* will vary from species to species and from tissue to tissue. For example, administration of *N*-OH-AAF to rats leads to formation of a DNA-adduct arising from an acetoxyarylamine metabolite formed by NOAT. In contrast, when *N*-OH-AAF is given to mice, it is deacetylated to form *N*-OH-AF which is then further metabolized to a reactive sulfate ester.

N-glucuronidation of *N*-hydroxyarylamines forms relatively stable metabolites at physiologic pH which are eliminated in the bile or renally. However, in the acidic milieu of urine, the *N*-glucuronides undergo acid hydrolysis releasing the free hydroxyarylamine which may further undergo protonation of the *N*-hydroxy group with a loss of water to form the highly reactive arylnitrenium ion. This is the metabolic pathway which is likely to be responsible for the induction of bladder cancer by aromatic amine compounds.

Studies in animals suggest that the NAT, NOAT and OAT activities reside on the same enzyme protein[11,12]. Although NOAT activity has not been clearly demonstrated to occur in humans, a close relationship between NAT and OAT activity has been observed[13,14]. Thus, NAT (which is generally thought to be involved in the generation of *inactive* metabolites) appears to play a dual role and with respect to carcinogenic arylamines also functions in the *activation* of these compounds.

The earliest evidence that NAT may play a role in the bioactivation of aromatic amines came from studies in dogs. Unlike humans, the dog is unable to acetylate arylamine carcinogens[15]. Studies showed that administration of acetylated arylamines to dogs resulted in urinary bladder and liver tumors, whereas only urinary bladder tumors were observed after administration of unacetylated arylamines[16]. These observations suggested that acetylation was important in the ontogeny of hepatic cancer but not of bladder cancer.

The data in dogs are also consistent with observations in humans where acetylator phenotype has been recognized as a risk factor in developing toxicity to arylamine compounds. In general, fast acetylators will show a higher degree of toxicity in those tissues which are closer to the site of administration of the arylamine carcinogen. This suggests that efficient *N*-acetylation may lead to *activation* of carcinogenic arylamine substrates which contributes to the development of, for example, colerectal cancer[17]. In contrast, slow acetylators appear to be at higher risk of developing cancers from these compounds at distant sites (sites of excretion) presumably because the dose of unacetylated parent compound reaching these tissues is higher in slow acetylators as compared to fast acetylators. These observations suggest that failure to *inactivate* carcinogenic arylamines by *N*-acetylation may play a role in the development of, for example, urinary bladder cancer[14].

The enzymes responsible for the *N*-acetylation of carcinogenic arylamines have recently been identified[18,19]. Although the NAT1 and NAT2 enzymes preferentially acetylate monomorphic and polymorphic substrates, respectively, the carcinogenic arylamine substrates do not fall into either category. Both the NAT1 and NAT2 forms of NAT are efficient in the acetylation of carcinogenic arylamine substrates. The actual identity of the enzyme involved in catalyzing OAT activity in humans remains to be determined.

The enzyme(s) involved in deacetylation are not well characterized. Deacetylation is an activity associated with a group of enzymes collectively known as carboxylesterases or nonspecific esterases. These enzymes are often referred to as serine hydrolases because they contain a serine group at their active site. Most of these enzymes also deacetylate arylamide compounds and are termed amidases or carboxylesterases/amidases. Multiple carboxylesterase isoenzymes which are capable of metabolizing a wide variety of carboxylic ester, aromatic amide and thioester substrates have been purified from rat liver[20,21]. Recently, an enzyme which catalyzes the deacetylation of AAF has also been purified from human liver. However, identity of this enzyme with the nonspecific esterases from other species has not been confirmed[22].

Deacetylation may play an important role in modulating the toxicity of carcinogenic arylamines. Microsomal deacetylation of both arylamides and arylhydroxamic acids has been shown to generate mutagenic products in several species *in vitro*[23,24]. Although *N*-OH-AAF itself is mutagenic, its deacetylated metabolite *N*-OH-AF has a much higher mutagenic activity[25,26]. In addition, administration of either AAF or *N*-OH-AAF to laboratory animals results in the formation of predominantly one, nonacetylated DNA-adduct (*N*-(deoxyguanosin-8-yl)-2-aminofluorene)[27,28]. It is generally assumed that the first step in the initiation of carcinogenesis and mutagenesis by 2-acetylaminofluorene (AAF) is *N*-hydroxylation. However, a study in rabbits showed that almost all of the mutagenic products of AAF metabolism in rabbit lung were initiated by deacetylation to AF and that

60% of the total hepatic metabolism of AAF to mutagenic products also required deacetylation of AAF to AF first, followed by *N*-hydroxylation[23]. The lack of NOAT activity towards *N*-OH-AAF in human liver cytosols suggests that activation of carcinogenic arylamides may proceed via pathways involving the deacetylated arylamine and hydroxyarylamine metabolites.

In addition to their carcinogenic and mutagenic effects, studies have shown that 2-aminofluorene (AF) and 2-acetylaminofluorene (AAF) are toxic to the embryos of laboratory animals in culture. Because embryotoxicity is not observed in the absence of a hepatic activating system, it is clear that these compounds require metabolic activation to exert their embryotoxic effects[29]. The profile of malformations produced when embryos were cultured with two metabolites of AAF (*N*-OH and *N*-acetoxy-AAF) was different from those observed when AAF was added to embryo culture in the presence of a hepatic activating system. These observations suggested that other metabolites were contributing to the observed dysmorphogenesis. Addition of reduced glutathione attenuated the embryotoxicity of *N*-acetoxy-AAF, thus further supporting the theory that reactive metabolites were responsible for the observed effects[30].

Further study revealed that ring hydroxylations were important in mediating the malformations produced by AAF. Although the ring-hydroxylated metabolites of AAF were thought to be inactive, 7-OH-AAF was shown to exert dysneurulatory effect on embryos in culture[31]. In this case, the proximate dysmorphogen is suggested to be the catechol metabolite 6,7-dihydroxy-AAF[32].

Deacetylation may also contribute to embryotoxicity. *N*-OH-AF produced malformations and embryolethality in the absence of an exogenous bioactivating system[33], whereas the deacetylated metabolite 7-OH-AF produced generalized embryotoxic and cytotoxic effects at concentrations 10-fold lower than 7-OH-AAF[34].

In addition to being toxic to embryos *in vitro*, AAF has been shown to be teratogenic in rats and mice when administered *in vivo*[35]. In this instance, a role for the placenta in bioactivation of carcinogenic arylamines might be suggested. However, the metabolism of these compounds by placenta has not been investigated thoroughly.

Placental biotransformation of arylamines

In a recent study we investigated the placental biotransformation of the carcinogenic arylamine AF and its acetylated arylamide metabolite, AAF.

Table 4.1. *Summary of the velocities and inhibition of 2-acetylaminofluorene (AAF) and p-nitrophenyl acetate (pNPA) deacetylation: Comparison of data obtained in human placenta and human liver*

			Placenta	Liver	
AAF	VELOCITY at 50 µM AAF	nmol/ min/mg	3.86 ± 0.37	5.94 ± 0.46	$p < 0.006$
	IC$_{50}$ of BPNPP	µM	1657 ± 106	6.06 ± 0.33	$p < 0.001$
	IC$_{50}$ of CEI INHIBITION	µM	37.4 ± 3.9	10.4 ± 7.4	$p < 0.001$
pNPA	VELOCITY at 500 µM pNPA	nmol/ min/mg	83.0 ± 6.7	2167 ± 57	$p < 0.001$
	IC$_{50}$ of BPNPP INHIBITION	µM	1719 ± 249	12.0 ± 4.1	$p < 0.001$
	IC$_{50}$ of CEI INHIBITION	µM	54.9 ± 9.3	10.4 ± 1.6	$p < 0.002$

Data shown are MEAN $\pm$ SEM; N = 6 (placenta); N = 5 (liver).
Statistical comparisons (placenta versus liver) were by non-paired t-test with a significance level of $p < 0.05$.

Because the oxidative metabolism of AAF by human placenta has previously been investigated, the study described in this chapter focused on the *N*-acetylation and deacetylation activity of human placental cytosol and microsomes respectively. The balance between these two activities in placenta may be important in determining what effect placental biotransformation reactions may have on mediating the exposure of the developing fetus to these potentially teratogenic compounds. For example, the bioactivated metabolites of arylamine compounds found in cigarette smoke may contribute to some of the adverse effects associated with smoking during pregnancy.

For this study, subcellular fractions of placental tissue were prepared following standard differential centrifugation techniques.

Inhibition of AAF deacetylation by placental microsomes was $30.0 \pm 1.87\%$ in contrast to the $93.8 \pm 0.88\%$ inhibition of hepatic activity. The IC$_{50}$ of BPNPP inhibition of AAF deacetylation was 1657 ± 106 μM for liver.

Table 4.1 is a summary of the human placental and liver deacetylation activities and their corresponding parameters of inhibition.

The role of the placenta in mediating the embryotoxicity of carcinogenic arylamines is not known, but based on the teratogenic effects observed *in vitro* and *in vivo* in laboratory animals, bioactivation of these compounds by placental enzymes may be important.

N-acetylation of 2-aminofluorence

The apparent affinity of *N*-acetylation of the arylamine substrate 2-aminofluorene (AF) by human placental cytosol has been shown to be similar to that measured for the partially purified NAT1 enzyme of human liver. The apparent affinity of AF acetylation by human liver NAT2 is an order of magnitude higher than that determined for NAT1 or for *N*-acetylation by placenta. These data suggest that the NAT activity of human placenta towards carcinogenic arylamines is predominantly attributable to NAT1, although the velocity of *N*-acetylation of these substrates in human placenta is similar to the activity in human liver.

Deacetylation of 2-acetylaminofluorene

Kinetic parameters of the deacetylation of the arylamide 2-acetylaminofluorene (AAF) by human placental or liver microsomes were not determined. Recent observations support the conclusion that the overall deacetylation activity observed is a composite of more than one (possibly several) enzyme activities, each with its own characteristic velocity and apparent affinity of deacetylation towards AAF. This conclusion has merit, given that most carboxylesterases are also active towards amide substrates[20,36,37].

Bis(4-nitrophenyl)phosphate (BPNPP) is an organophosphate compound which is a specific, active-site directed inhibitor of carboxylesterase enzymes[38]. Under physiologic conditions, the enzyme inhibition is irreversible[39]. The profile of inhibition of AAF deacetylation by BPNPP in human liver microsomes compared to human placental microsomes shows striking differences. The estimated IC_{50} for inhibition of placental AAF deacetylation was almost 300 times higher than that determined for liver. Because individual carboxylesterases (purified from rat liver) show marked differences in their sensitivity to inhibition by BPNPP, the observed differences between placenta and liver are consistent with a difference in the profile of carboxylesterase enzymes between these two human tissues[39,40].

Chloroethyl isocyanate (CEI) is a degradation product of the antitumor drug carmustine (1,3-bis(2-chlorethyl)-1-nitrosourea; BCNU)[41]. Alkyl isocyanate compounds are highly reactive and will react with a variety of moieties such as amino, sulfhydryl, imidazole and carboxyl groups[42]. In addition, studies with chymotrypsin and elastase revealed that enzyme inactivation by alkyl isocyanates was a result of carbamoxylation of a serine at the active site[42,43]. The data in Table 4.1 show that CEI is effective in inhibiting both the hepatic and placental deacetylase enzymes, although inhibition of the placental activity still requires significantly higher inhibitor concentrations.

One possible explanation for the differences in enzyme inactivation between liver and placenta may lie in differences in the membrane milieu in which the enzyme activity resides. For this reason, any significant differences between liver and placental microsomes in accessibility of the inhibitor to the active site would probably be reflected by a much larger difference in IC_{50}. These observations may point to important differences between placenta and liver in the characteristics of the enzyme(s) involved in AAF deacetylation.

Deacetylation of p-*nitrophenyl acetate*

p-Nitrophenyl acetate (*p*NPA) is a prototype substrate for the carboxylesterase enzymes. It is metabolized by all five isoenzymes purified from rat liver, although the velocity of deacetylation between the different enzyme proteins varies from 5 to 130 μmol/min/mg purified enzyme protein[20,36,39].

A comparison of the deacetylation activity of placental and liver microsomes towards pNPA shows a remarkable contrast when compared to the relative activities between the two tissues towards AAF. In terms of absolute velocity of deacetylation, both the placental and liver enzymes had higher activities towards pNPA as a substrate than AAF. However, the hepatic enzymes preferentially deacetylate the carboxylester substrate rather than the amide substrate whereas the degree of difference in deacetylation velocity by placental microsomes towards the two substrates is not as great. These data lend further support to the hypothesis that the characteristics of the liver and placental enzymes are different.

Studies of microsomal AAF metabolism in rabbit[23] show certain similarities between the placental deacetylase activity and that of another extrahepatic tissue (lung). For example, rabbit hepatic deacetylase activity towards pNPA is five times higher than pulmonary activity. A similar difference between hepatic and placental activities was observed in the current study, although the extent of the difference was dependent on the substrate concentration.

Differential sensitivities to inhibitors was also observed in rabbit hepatic versus pulmonary deacetylase activities[23]. The highly reactive phosphorylating agent paraoxon inhibits both hepatic and pulmonary AAF metabolism to a similar extent. In contrast, pulmonary AAF deacetylation (which is inhibited greater than 90% by paraoxon) is only inhibited by 17% by 500 μM BPNPP. These data bear a striking similarity to the characteristics of placental AAF deacetylation which was maximally inhibited by 86.9 $\pm$ 3.1% by CEI but only 20.7 $\pm$ 3.6% at 500 /mu/M BPNPP. Nevertheless, several characteristics of the human placental deacetylase activity differ markedly from those of the lung. For example, BPNPP effectively inhibited the pulmonary deacetylation of pNPA, an inhibition which was not observed for placenta. Thus, in spite of several similarities, the characteristics of the enzyme activities of these two extrahepatic tissues are quite different.

Human deacetylase

Recently, an AAF deacetylase activity was purified from human liver[22]. The characteristics of this purified enzyme were compared to carboxylesterase enzymes from four other species. Several differences between the human enzyme and those of laboratory animals were noted. Although the majority of carboxylesterase enzymes characterized thus far have molecular weights ranging from 60 to 75 kD, the human AAF–DAC enzyme was identified as a 45 kD protein. Other purified human liver esterase activities also show molecular weights in the 60 kD range[20]. However, these activities may represent different enzymes, since the deacetylation of AAF was not tested with these 60 kD proteins.

A comparison of the N-terminal amino acid sequence (119 amino acids) of the purified human enzyme showed no homology to the N-terminal sequences of rat, rabbit, hamster or monkey carboxylesterases. In addition, the human enzyme did not contain the active site sequence motif which is common to serine hydrolases. These observations suggest that the human enzyme active in AAF deacetylation may not belong to the carboxylesterase/ amidase family of enzymes. However, a proven positive correlation between hepatic AAF deacetylation and pNPA deacetylation does suggest a relationship between these two DAC activities.

Oxidative metabolism of AAF

The hydroxylation of AAF has been studied previously in both human and primate tissues. The study showed that the placental microsomes contained enzyme activities capable of catalyzing both *N*-hydroxylations and ring hydroxylations of AAF, although the enzymes responsible for the observed activity were not identified. In human liver, the cytochrome P450 species implicated in the *N*-hydroxylation of carcinogenic arylamines in human liver is CYP1A2[44] whereas more than one form of cytochrome P450 appears to be involved in the ring hydroxylations of AAF[45].

An indication as to the identity of the enzyme(s) involved in the oxidative metabolism of AAF by human placenta is given by the observation that the AAF *N*-hydroxylating and ring-hydroxylating activities were significantly higher in placental microsomes taken from smoking mothers compared to nonsmoking mothers. Thus, CYP1A1, which is so highly induced in human placenta by smoking[46], may be the enzyme responsible for catalyzing the increased AAF *N*-hydroxylation activity observed in placentas from smoking mothers.

The major hydroxylated metabolite of AAF formed by placental microsomes was 7-OH-AAF[47] an observation which is also true for human liver[48]. This observation is of toxicologic interest since the 7-OH metabolite of AAF has been implicated in causing abnormal neurulation in embryos exposed to this metabolite in culture[32]. A positive correlation between 7-hydroxylation of AAF and 3-hydroxylation of benzo[a]pyrene (BP) suggests that these activities may be catalyzed by the same enzyme, possibly CYP1A1[49]. In contrast, the increased *N*-hydroxylation of AAF observed with smoking did not correlate with the oxidation of BP. Thus, in addition to CYP1A1, other enzymes may be involved in the oxidative metabolism of AAF in human placenta.

Studies in laboratory animals show that embryos transplacentally exposed to polycyclic armoatic hydrocarbon (PAH) inducers of CYP1A activity (3-methylcholanthrene) show an increased incidence in malformations when subsequently cultured with AAF[50]. Pre-exposure transplacentally to phenobarbital (PB) was without significant effect. These data indicate that induction of embryonic enzymes by PAH inducers enhances bioactivation of AAF to toxic and reactive metabolites. By analogy, placental enzymes are also sensitive to PAH inducers but not to PB induction, suggesting that the placenta may play an important role in mediating the embryotoxic effects of carcinogenic arylamines.

With respect to smoking, epidemiologic data indicate that smoking increases the risk of developing bladder cancer and the urine of smokers has been shown to be mutagenic[51]. Because cigarette smoke is known to contain significant levels of aromatic amines, the increased risk of bladder cancer with smoking is likely to be related to increased exposure to these compounds.

Fetuses are transplacentally exposed to carcinogenic arylamines found in cigarette smoke and in the environment. A study in which 4-aminobiphenyl hemoglobin (Hb) adducts were measured in fetuses of smoking and nonsmoking mothers presented evidence that these compounds not only cross the placenta but are also bioactivated *in utero* in humans[52]. Because the placental enzyme activities which function in the metabolism of carcinogenic arylamines and arylamides are induced by the PAHs found in cigarette smoke, placental metabolism of these compounds may have important toxicologic implicatons for the fetus.

Although 4-aminobiphenyl Hb adduct concentrations were always higher in the blood of smoking mothers compared to nonsmoking mothers, only half of the fetuses of smokers had adduct concentrations higher than those measured in fetuses of nonsmokers. These data might suggest that increased placental enzyme activity *decreased* the exposure of some fetuses to the arylamine compound by bioactivating the xenobiotic and intercepting it before it reached the fetus. Alternatively, a positive correlation between fetal 4-aminobiphenyl Hb adduct concentrations and maternal adduct concentrations suggests that the placenta may have *contributed* to *fetotoxicity* by transferring to the fetus the procarcinogenic/mutagenic metabolites which were further converted to their highly reactive forms by fetal enzymes.

Summary and conclusion

Recent studies reveal some characteristics of the placental enzymes involved in the metabolism of carcinogenic arylamines and suggest some important toxicologic implications of placental arylamine metabolism. Perhaps the most important observation is that the placenta contains the enzymes implicated in the metabolism of carcinogenic arylamines to their toxic, reactive forms. Both NAT and DAC activity towards AF and AAF, respectively, proceed with an apparent affinity and velocity similar to that observed for human liver. The balance between these two activities may determine whether the net effect of placental metabolism is toxification or detoxification. For example, although 7-OH-AAF is embryotoxic, its deacetylated metabolite 7-OH-AF shows embryotoxicity at significantly lower concentrations. In this instance, a high NAT to DAC activity ratio would be advantageous. Nevertheless, because dysmorphogenesis by 7-OH-AFF is so specific (targeted to the neural tube), a high NAT activity would be undesirable, especially if the embryotoxic agent (AF or AAF) is given at the stage of embryonic neural tube formation.

The examples given above underscore the importance of understanding all aspects of placental xenobiotic metabolism. Although the *N*-acetylation activity of human placenta is similar to human liver, the characteristics of DAC activity in these two human tissues is vastly different. Based on current knowledge, it is clear that conclusions drawn from data obtained in one tissue (e.g., liver) cannot be extrapolated to another tissue (e.g., placenta), even within the same species.

The data presented in this chapter show that the pathways for activating carcinogenic arylamines are present in human placenta. However, the *net* effect these placental bioactivation reactions will have on the developing fetus will ultimately depend on the balance between activating and detoxifying pathways in both placental and fetal tissues.

The placenta plays a critical role in mammalian development. Failure of the placenta to transport all the nutrients required by the growing embryo/fetus results in, at best, some degree of developmental retardation and at worst, an adverse pregnancy outcome. On the other hand, the inability of the placenta to exclude harmful substances, and to selectively transport only those elements required by the fetus, is the cornerstone of the discipline of teratology.

Although it is true that enzyme activities measured in term placenta may not reflect the activities present during organogenesis, even low levels of activity may activate a potentially teratogenic molecule to a highly reactive metabolite. Covalent binding of a reactive intermediate with a critical cell target in a rapidly differentiating system such as the embryo, may ultimately be manifested as teratogenicity. On the other hand, metabolic activation of carcinogenic compounds at term may have important postnatal consequences which do not manifest themselves immediately but become apparent several years after birth as developmental toxicity (e.g., neurotoxicity) or carcinogenesis.

Footnote: This has been supported by a grant from MRC, Canada.

References

1. Hoffman D, Hecht SS: Advances in tobacco carcinogenesis. In *Chemical Carcinogenesis and Mutagenesis* I (Cooper CS, Grover PL eds.) Springer-Verlag, Berlin, 1990, pp. 63–102.
2. Bjeldanes LF, Morris MM, Felton JS, Healy SK, Stuermer DH, Berry T, Timourian H, Hatch FT: Mutagens from the cooking of food. II. Survey by Ames/*Salmonella* test of mutagen formation in the major protein-rich foods of the American diet. *Food Chem Toxicol* 1982; 20: 357–63.
3. Felton JS, Knize MG: Heterocyclic-amine mutagens/carcinogens in foods. In *Chemical Carcinogenesis and Mutagenesis* I (Cooper CS, Grover PL, eds.) 1990, pp. 471–502; Springer-Verlag, Berlin.
4. Doll R, Peto R: The causes of cancer: Quantitative estimates of avoidable risk of cancer in the United States today. *J Natl Cancer Inst* 1981; 66: 1191–308.

5. Rehn L: Blasengeschwulste bei Fuschin-Arbeitern. *Arch Klin Chir* 1895; 50: 588–600.
6. Hueper WC, Wiley FH, Wolfe HD: Experimental production of bladder tumors in dogs by administration of beta-naphthylamine. *J Indian Hyg Toxicol* 1938; 20: 46–84.
7. Parkes HG, Evans AEJ: Epidemiology of aromatic amine cancers. In *Chemical Carcinogens*. (Searle CE, ed.) American Chemical Society Monograph 182, 1984, pp. 277–301, Washington DC.
8. Miller EC: Some current perspectives on chemical carcinogenesis: presidential address. *Cancer Res* 1978; 38: 1479–96.
9. Kadlubar FF, Hammons GJ: The role of cytochrome P-450 in the metabolism of chemical carcinogens. In *Mammalian Cytochromes P-450*. (Guengerich FP, ed.) 1987, pp. 81–130, CRC Press, Boca Raton.
10. Lotikar PD: Enzymatic *N*-hydroxylation of aromatic amides. In *Biological Oxidation of Nitrogen in Organic Molecules* (Gorrod JW, Damani LA, eds.) 1985, pp. 163–174, Ellis Horwood Ltd., Chichester.
11. Saito K, Shinohara A, Kamataki T: *N*-hydroxyarylamine *O*-acetyltransferase in hamster liver: identity with arylhydroxamic acid *N,O*-acetyltransferase and arylamine *N*-acetyltransferase. *J Biochem* 1986; 99: 1689–97.
12. Trinidad A, Hein DW, Rustan TD, Ferguson RJ, Miller LS, Bucher KD, Kirlin WG, Ogolla F, Andrews AF: Purification of hepatic polymorphic arylamine *N*-acetyltransferase from homozygous rapid acetylator inbred hamster: identity with polymorphic *N*-hydroxyarylamine-*O*-acetyltransferase. *Cancer Res* 1990; 50: 7942–9.
13. Flammang TJ, Yamazoe Y, Guengerich FP, Kadlubar FF: The *S*-acetylcoenzyme A-dependent metabolic activation of the carcinogoen *N*-hydroxy-2-aminofluorene by human liver cytosol and its relationship to the aromatic amine *N*-acetyltransferase phenotype. *Carcinogenesis* 1987; 8: 1967–70.
14. Kirlin WG, Trinidad A, Yerokun T, Ogolla F, Ferguson RJ, Andrews AF, Brady PK, Hein DW: Polymorphic expression of acetyl coenzyme A-dependent arylamine *N*-acetyltransferase and acetyl coenzyme A-dependent *O*-acetyltransferase-mediated activation of *N*-hydroxyarylamines by human bladder cytosol. *Cancer Res* 1989; 49: 2448–54.
15. Williams RT: Comparative patterns of drug metabolism. *Federation Proc* 1967; 26: 1029–39.
16. Poirier LA, Miller JA, Miller EC: The *N* and ring hydroxylation of 2-acetylaminofluorene and the failure to detect *N*-acetylation of 2-aminofluorene in the dog. *Cancer Res* 1963; 23: 790–800.
17. Kirlin WG, Ogolla F, Andrews AF, Trinidad A, Ferguson RJ, Yerokun T, Mpezo M, Hein DW: Acetylator genotype-dependent expression of arylamine *N*-acetyltransferase in human colon cytosol from non-cancer and colorectal cancer patients. *Cancer Res* 1991; 51: 549–55.
18. Grant DM, Blum M, Beer M, Meyer UA: Monomorphic and polymorphic human arylamine *N*-acetyltransferases: a comparison of liver isozymes and expressed products of two cloned genes. *Mol Pharmacol* 1991; 39: 184–91.
19. Grant DM, Lottspeich F, Meyer UA: Evidence for two closely related isozymes of arylamine *N*-acetyltransferase in human liver. *FEBS Lett* 1989; 244: 203–7.
20. Heymann E: Carboxylesterases and amidases. In *Enzymatic Basis of Detoxication* (Jakoby WB, ed.) 1980, pp. 291–232, Academic Press Inc, New York.

21. Mentlein R, Schumann M, Heymann E: Comparative chemical and immunological characterization of five lipolytic enzymes (carboxylesterases) from rat liver microsomes. *Arch Biochem Biophys* 1984; 234: 612–21.
22. Probst MR, Jeno P, Meyer USA: Purification and characterization of a human liver arylacetamide deacetylase. *Biochem Biophys Res Commun* 1991; 177: 453–9.
23. Aune T, Vanderslice RR, Croft JE, Dybing E, Bend JR, Philpot RM: Deacetylation to 2-aminofluorene as a major initial reaction in the microsomal metabolism of 2-acetylaminofluorene to mutagenic products in preparations from rabbit lung and liver. *Cancer Res* 1985; 45: 5859–66.
24. Kaneda S, Seno T, Takeishi K: Main pathway for mutagenic activation of 2-acetylaminofluorene by guinea pig liver homogenates. *Biochem Biophys Res Commun* 1979; 90: 750–6.
25. McCaman MW, Robins E: Fluorimetric method for the determination of phenylalanine in serum. *J Lab Clin Med* 1962; 59: 885–90.
26. Schut HA, Wirth PJ, Thorgeirsson SS: Mutagenic activation of *N*-hydroxy-2-acetylaminofluorene in the *Salmonella* test system: the role of deacetylation by liver and kidney fractions from mouse and rat. *Mol Pharmacol* 1978; 14: 682–92.
27. Beland FA, Kadlubar FF: Metabolic activation and DNA adducts of aromatic amines and nitroaromatic hydrocarbons. In *Chemical Carcinogenesis and Mutagenesis* I (Cooper CS, Grover PL, eds.) 1990, pp. 267–325, Springer-Verlag, Berlin.
28. Poirer MC, Hunt JM, True B, Laishes BA, Young JF, Beland FA: DNA adduct formation, removal and persistence in rat liver during one month feeding of 2-acetylaminofluorene. *Carcinogenesis* 1984; 5: 1591–6.
29. Faustman-Watts EM, Yang HL, Namkung MJ, Greenaway JC, Fantel AG, Juchau MR: Mutagenic, cytotoxic and teratogenic effects of 2-acetylaminofluorene and reactive metablites *in vitro*. *Teratogen Carcinogen Mutagen* 1984a; 4: 273–83.
30. Faustman-Watts EM, Namkung MJ, Juchau MR: Modulation of the embryotoxicity *in vitro* of reactive metabolies of 2-acetylaminofluorene by reduced glutathione and ascorbate and via sulfation. *Toxicol Appl Pharmacol* 1986; 86: 400–10.
31. Faustman-Watts EM, Greenaway JC, Namkung MJ, Fantel AG, Juchau MR: Teratogencitiy *in vitro* of two deacetylated metabolies of *N*-hydroxy-2-acetylaminofluorene. *Toxicol Appl Pharmacol* 1984b; 76: 161–71.
32. Harris C, Stark KL, Luchtel DL, Juchau MR: Abnormal neurulation induced by 7-hydroxy-2-acetylaminofluorene and acetaminophen: evidence of catechol metabolites as proximate dysmorphogens. *Toxicol Appl Pharmacol* 1989; 101: 432–46.
33. Faustman-Watts EM, Greenaway JC, Namkung MJ, Fantel AG, Juchau MR: Teratogenicity *in vitro* of 2-acetylaminofluorene: role of biotransformation in the rat. *Teratology* 1983; 27: 19–28.
34. Stark KL, Harris C, Juchau MR: Modulation of the embryotoxicity and cytotoxicity elicited by 7-hydroxy-2-acetylaminofluorene and acetaminophen via deacetylation. *Toxicol Appl Pharmacol* 1989; 97: 548–60.
35. Juchau MR: Bioactivation in chemical teratogenesis. *Ann Rev Pharmacol Toxicol* 1989; 29: 165–87.
36. Heymann E, Mentlein R: Carboxylesterases–amidases. In *Methods in Enzymology* (Colowick SP, Sidney P, eds.) 1981, pp. 333–344, Academic Press, New York.
37. Heymann E, Mentlein R, Rix H: Hydrolysis of aromatic amides as assay for

carboxylesterases–amidases. In *Methods in Enzymology* 1981, pp. 405–409, Academic Press, New York.

38. Heymann E, and Krisch K: Phosphorsaure-bis(*p*-nitrophenylester), ein neur Hemmstoff mikrosomaler carboxylesterasen. *Hoppe-Seyler's Z Physiol Chem* 1967; 348: 609–19.

39. Mentlein R, Suttorp M, Heymann E: Specificity of purified monoaceylglycerol lipase, palmitoyl-CoA hydrolase, palmitoyl-carnitine hydrolase, and non-specific carboxylesterase from rat liver microsomes. *Arch Biochem Biophys* 1984; 228: 230–46.

40. Heymann E, Krisch K, Buch H, Buzello W: Inhibition of phenacetin- and acetanilide-induced methemoglobinemia in the rat by the carboxylesterase inhibitor bis-[*p*-nitrophenyl] phosphate. *Biochem Pharmacol* 1969; 18: 801–11.

41. Calabresi P, Chabner BA: Antineoplastic agents. In *The Pharmacological Basis of Therapeutics, Eighth Edition* (Goodman Gilman A, Rall TW, Nies AS, Taylor P, ed.) 1990, pp. 1209–1263, Pergamon Press, New York.

42. Brown WE, Wold F: Alkyl isocyanates as active-site-specific reagents for serine proteases. Identification of the active-site serine as the site of reaction. *Biochemistry* 1973; 12: 835–40.

43. Babson JR, Reed DJ, Sinkey MA: Active site specific inactivation of chymotrypsin by cyclohexyl isocyanate formed during degradation of the carcinostatic 1-(2-chloroethyl)-3-cyclohexyl-1-nitrosourea. *Biochemistry* 1977; 16: 1584–9.

44. Butler MA, Iwasaki M, Guengerich FP, Kadlubar FF: Human cytochrome P-450P (P-4501A2), the phenacetin *O*-deethylase, is primarily responsible for the hepatic 3-demethylation of caffeine and N-oxidation of carcinogenic arylamines. *Proc Natl Acad Sci USA* 1989; 86: 7696–700.

45. McManus ME: The role of cytochromes P-450 and N-acetyl transferase in the carcinogenicity of aromatic amines and amides. *Clin Exp Pharmacol Physiol* 1989; 16: 491–5.

46. Pasanen M, Pelkonen O: Human placental xenobiotic and steroid biotransformations catalyzed by cytochromes P450, epoxide hydrolase, and glutathione *S*-transferase activities and their relationship to maternal cigarette smoking. *Drug Metab Rev* 1989–90; 21: 427–61.

47. Juchau MR, Namkung MJ, Berry DL, Zachariah PK: Oxidative biotransformation of 2-acetylaminofluorene in fetal and placental tissues of humans and monkeys: correlations with aryl hydrocarbon hydroxylase activities. *Drug Metab Dispos* 1975; 3: 494–501.

48. McManus ME, Minchin RF, Wirth PJ, Thorgeirsson SS: Kinetic evidence for the involvement of multiple forms of human cytochrome P-450 in the metabolism of 2-acetylaminofluorene. *Carcinogenesis* 1983; 4: 693–7.

49. Pasanen M, Haaparanta T, Sundin M, Sivonen P, Vahakangas K, Raunio H, Hines R, Gustafsson JA, Pelkonen O: Immunochemical and molecular biological studies on human placental cigarette smoke-inducible cytochrome P450-dependent monooxygenase activities. *Toxicology* 1990; 62: 175–87.

50. Juchau MR, Giachelli CM, Fantel AG, Greenaway JC, Shepard TH, Faustman-Watts EM: Effects of 3-methylcholanthrene and phenobarbital on the capacity of embryos to bioactivate teratogens during organogenesis. *Toxicol Appl Pharmacol* 1985; 80: 137–46.

51. Evans DAP: *N*-Acetyltransferase. *Pharmacol Ther* 1989; 42: 157–234.

52. Coghlin J, Gann PH, Hammond SK, Skipper PL, Taghizadeh K, Paul M, Tannenbaum SR: 4-Aminobiphenyl hemoglobin adducts in fetuses exposed to the tobacco smoke carcingoen *in utero*. *J Natl Cancer Inst* 1991; 83: 274–80.

5
Antepartum fetal monitoring in the oncologic patient

Y. EZRA AND K. PANTER

Introduction

In this chapter we consider fetal monitoring in pregnancies in women with cancer where a decision has been made to continue the pregnancy to the third trimester to achieve fetal viability. These cases are beyond the "dilemma phase" of the first and second trimester. The general principles of fetal monitoring would apply also to pregnancies where the malignancy is in the fetus, but the specific management of such cases is discussed elsewhere. This chapter serves as a brief overview of fetal monitoring, not for the perinatologist but for health care professionals from the other disciplines involved in the management of such patients.

These pregnancies are considered "high risk" because of the maternal condition, which may affect the fetus through the maternal systemic effects of malignancy (e.g., malnutrition and pyrexial illness), the effects of investigation and diagnosis (X-ray, thyroid radionucleotide and bone scans), the effects of treatment (e.g., surgery, anesthesia, chemotherapy, radiotherapy, hormonal therapy and analgesia), or direct effects of the maternal tumor on the fetus by the hormone secretion and, rarely, trans-placental metastasis.

Fetal lung maturity is usually expected after the 34th week of pregnancy in the majority of babies (diabetic mothers' fetuses are an exception because of delayed fetal lung maturity), but the course of the disease in either mother or fetus may necessitate earlier delivery before lung maturity has been achieved. When premature delivery is planned prior to 34 weeks' gestation, corticosteroids should be given at least 24 hours beforehand, to decrease the risk of respiratory distress syndrome (RDS) in the newborn.

The route of delivery would be influenced by both maternal and fetal factors and must be assessed on an individual basis. Anatomical distortion of the vaginal/vulvar or the perineal area (e.g., after vulvar irradiation or radical vulvectomy) may make abdominal delivery preferable. Conization of the cervix may result in both cervical incompetence and cervical stenosisis but is not usually an indication for cesarean section *per se*. Cesarean delivery may be indicated when there is any evidence of remaining invasive disease (not a CIN state), or if disorders of cervical dilation during labor prevent progress. Intra-abdominal and pelvic tumors (even benign) may prevent engagement of the fetal head and this may disrupt the descent of the presenting part through the birth canal.

Biochemical parameters

Hormone levels have been used in the past to monitor placental function in an attempt to assess fetal well-being. Today, they are not in clinical use. The most common hormones were E3 (estriol) and hPL (human placental lactogen). Estriol is produced jointly by of the maternal adrenals, the placenta, and the fetal adrenals and liver. The level of E3 was found to have a very large range when measured during pregnancy and a low level of E3 was not necessarily indicative of fetal compromise. The current use of E3 levels is as part of the "'triple screen" during the second trimester to assess the risk of Down's syndrome in the fetus.

hPL is a hormone produced by the placenta and has been found to be an even less accurate predictor of fetal well-being. Its use today has been largely abandoned.

Fetal movements

Fetal activity *in utero* is a sign of fetal well-being, and from this arose the concept of monitoring fetal movement to investigate the fetal condition[1-6]. The first maternal sensation of fetal movement usually occurs at between 16 and 20 weeks' gestation. It starts as an infrequent, weak "butterfly-like" flickering which gradually increases in frequency and intensity. During the first part of the second trimester it may sometimes be impossible to differentiate fetal movement from intestinal activity, but as pregnancy progresses the movements are more apparent to the pregnant woman.

The daily average number of fetal movements in a normal pregnancy is approximately 200 during the 20th week, increasing to more than 500 by the 32nd week of pregnancy; the individual variation might be expected to range from 50 to 950. In multifetal pregnancy the daily number might be expected to be higher. A normal "physiological" movement free period may be up to 75 minutes in duration[7]. With ultrasound it is possible to see all fetal movement but a mother usually recognises only about 80% of them. Maternal sensation of the fetal movements may be diminished if the placenta is located anteriorly or if there is polyhydramnios. There are some CNS malformations that may be associated with a true decrease in fetal movement, as well as the muscular dystrophies.

If a fetus is in a compromised state, fetal movements usually gradually decrease in number and intensity until fetal death occurs. "High risk" pregnancies complicated by preeclampsia, diabetes mellitus, maternal renal disease, rhesus isoimmunization, etc. may be associated with both a subjective and objective decrease in fetal movement which is thought to reflect the fetal response to hypoxia and other stresses. The sequence of events begins usually with weakening of fetal movement and only later do they cease completely. A decrease in the frequency of movement without a change in their intensity is not generally a worrying sign and may assist us in differentiating between a temporary, physiological decrease and a pathological decrease in association with fetal distress prior to fetal demise. Fetal activity of less than three movements per hour or the complete cessation of movement during any 12-hour period is termed a "movement alarm signal" (MAS), and was found by Sadovsky *et al*[8] to be very useful in the management of high-risk pregnancies associated with specific pathologic conditions[1–3,6]. The association of decreased fetal activity and hypoxia was shown in sheep models, when a mild decrease in oxygen tension was associated with cessation of fetal limb movement[7].

The existence of fetal movement is reassuring evidence of fetal well-being, but their absence demands further evaluation to determine whether fetal compromise is the cause of the decreased activity.

There are several reported methods of maternal "kick-counting" that differ very slightly although they are, in principle, identical. Kick counting is valuable only after the 25th week of gestation when one would consider acting upon a poor result (prior to this gestational age the fetus can seldom survive out of the uterine cavity). It should be performed three times daily over a 30-minute period (Fig. 5.1). If four or more movements are encountered within 30 minutes the woman can stop counting until the next period of the day. If less than four movements were noticed, she should continue to count for another one, two and up to four hours until she feels the fetal movements as usual. If more than ten movements were felt during the 4-hour period, she can stop until the next counting period. The sensation of fetal movements may be decreased during maternal activity and lying position on the left side may aid the perception of normal fetal movement. The kick-count method has a 21% false positive rate. Within

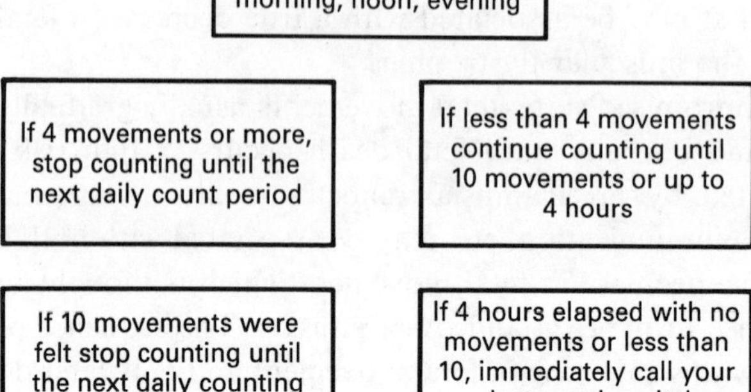

Fig. 5.1   High-risk daily movements count.

the framework of hospital-based fetal monitoring diminished fetal movement is not the first sign for fetal compromise (contrast stress test will usually be disturbed before the movements will be decreased), but for the majority of women at home this is the only obstetrical "test" readily available.

Electronic fetal heart rate monitoring

Recording of the fetal heart rate is done using an electronic monitor based on the Doppler ultrasound principle. The same instrument can give also some information about uterine contractions if there are any at the time of performing the test.

The woman can be lying or seated on a comfortable chair provided she is tilted to the left in order to avoid supine hypotension[13]. The transducer is then placed on the maternal abdomen and the fetal heart rate is automatically calculated and presented as a mean of the last three beats. This is represented visually as a graph drawn continuously on paper, at a rate of between 1 and 3 cm per minute. This enables the observer to evaluate the fetal heart pattern on a time-based scale. A specific device (event marker) is used to allow the woman to mark the same paper graph whenever she feels a fetal movement. Another transducer which is pressure sensitive may be applied to the mother's abdomen in the fundal area, to provide a qualitative, temporal record of uterine contractions. This recording is displayed on the same paper but as a different line, in parallel to the fetal heart rate recording.

Electronic fetal monitoring (EFM) may be tested as an nonstress test (NST) or as a contraction stress test (CST), as the NST is performed when there are no uterine contractions, and the CST assists in evaluating the fetal heart activity in the presence of uterine contractions, either spontaneous or intentionally evoked for specific indications.

NST (nonstress test)

This test is performed without concurrent external stimulation or uterine contractions. The baseline fetal heart rate should normally range between 120 and 160 beats per minute (bpm). The normal beat to beat variation (between the QRS complexes) which is called the short-term variability (STV), cannot be recorded by the external ultrasonic device (which provides an *average* value over the last three beats), but may be seen by using an internal electrode that is attached to the presenting fetal part (this can be done only during labor when the membranes are ruptured). The long-term variability (LTV) should be observed using the external abdominal monitor, and this is presented as 2–6 waveform-like fluctuations per minute, with an amplitude of 5–25 bpm. Temporary accelerations are usually observed during the pregnancy and they increase in amplitude according to the development and maturation of the fetal sympathetic nervous system. These accelerations are considered to represent a fetal response to various stimuli such as self-movements, external vibrations, loud noise, and uterine contractions[6]. After 30 weeks, we expect to see at least two accelerations in a 20-minute period. These accelerations should have an amplitude of more than 15 bpm above the baseline, and be at least 15 seconds in duration. Before 33 weeks, lower amplitude accelerations may be seen. The presence of accelerations in the recording is essential for the definition of the NST as "reactive" (reassuring).

There are certain conditions under which accelerations may not be observed. During normal fetal sleep, which can last 20–40 minutes, there are usually no accelerations. If no accelerations are observed during a 20-minute trace, the test should be continued for another 20 minutes. Some medications such as narcotics, phenobarbital, and beta-blockers may also be associated with a temporary absence of accelerations[9,10]. Chronic smoking is also associated with decreased placental perfusion and less accelerations[11]. In addition, it has been reported that a healthy term fetus may not demonstrate accelerations for prolonged periods of time, even up to 80 minutes. In most cases, however, one or no accelerations in a 40-minute period is considered as a "nonreactive" test and should be managed as such until proven otherwise. The false positive results of a nonreactive NST may be as high as 60–75%, and some claim even higher[13]. Since most of the fetal accelerations are associated with fetal movements, some consider the simultaneous marking of movements by the mother as futile. Variable declarations may be seen during a normal NST, and if mild in nature (less than 20 bpm in amplitude, or last less than 20 seconds), they may be ignored if normal accelerations are present[15], and the trace fulfils the other criteria of normality. The false negative rates of the NST may be higher in high-risk pregnancies such as maternal diabetes and fetal intrauterine growth restriction (IUGR)[16,17], and in these cases NST should be performend *at least* twice weekly or even daily, with other tests such as the biophysical profile and CST. The fetal heart rate trace can be considered to be a "snapshot" of the fetus which reflects fetal well-being at the time of the test, but cannot be extrapolated to provide any inference about the fetal condition subsequent to that time.

CST (contraction stress test)

This test was conceived to assist in the evaluation of the feto-placental oxygen reserve. This *reserve* is normally always present in a *normal* fetus but shows a physiological decrease as pregnancy progresses and the ageing placenta supports an enlarging fetus. Uterine contraction is associated with the cessation of the flow of blood between the chorionic villi; this causes a cessation in the feto-maternal gas exchange with a transient relative fetal hypoxia. In a normal healthy fetus, its oxygen *reserve* is able to support it during uterine contractions, however if this is not the case it will be manifest by a temporary bradycardia on the EFM. Such decreases in feto-placental reserve is often seen in conjunction with maternal pre-eclampsia and intrauterine growth retardation.

The duration of this test is 1–2 hours. The woman should be lying in the semi-fowler position. After baseline recording of the fetal heart rate for 15–20 minutes, if there are at least three spontaneous uterine contractions in a 10-minute period the behavior of the fetal rate and temporal association of any observed changes should be evaluated carefully. If there are no spontaneous contractions, or less than three per 10 minutes, an intravenous infusion of oxytocin should be instituted until that contraction frequency is achieved. The concentration of oxytocin used is 10 milliunits in 1 liter of normal saline and the dose is increased using the IVAC starting at 1–2 mU per minute and increasing by 1–2 mU increments every 20–30 minutes. Another method for evoking uterine contraction is by nipple stimulation which results in the production of endogenous oxytocin from the neurohypophysis.

Contraindications for the OCT include suspected preterm labor or a history of previous preterm labor, placenta previa, polyhydramnios, multifetal gestation, premature rupture of membranes (PROM), and a previous classical caesarian section.

Evaluation of the test results

A negative test is reported when there are no late decelerations in the presence of three uterine contractions over a 10-minute test. A positive test is reported when there is a late deceleration after each of the contractions in a 10-minute test. A suspicious test is reported if there are late decelerations after some, but *not* after every contraction. An unsatisfactory test is reported if there are less than three contractions per 10 minutes or if the technical quality of the tracing is reduced. Hyperstimulation of the uterus is defined when there is more than one contraction every 2 minutes, and late decelerations may be considered not to reflect either a chronic or acute decrease in the utero-placental blood flow.

The false negative incidence of the CST is quite low, but the false positive rate may be as high as 45–50%. A negative test may be reassuring for a period of one week[17]. A positive test is *not* an indication for immediate cesarean section, and other tests such as frequent serial NST and/or BPP may be performed in order to corroborate the positive CST result. A suspicious or equivocal CST should be repeated within 24 hours.

Ultrasound

Ultrasound was first used to visualize the human fetus in the early 1960s. Since then there has been a huge improvement both in the technology and availability of real time two-dimensional ultrasound to visualize the fetus and its intrauterine environment. Whilst the perinatal benefits of routine ultrasound in a low-risk obstetric population have recently been questioned in a large North American study[19], its role in the management of high-risk pregnancies is undisputed. Conceptually, by visualizing the fetus in its intrauterine environment, ultrasound has enabled the perinatologist to perform a "physical examination" of the fetus *in utero*.

The applications of ultrasound in a high risk pregnancy

- Accurate dating of pregnancy
- Serial growth assessment

- Anatomical survey
- Assessment of placenta (site, architecture)
- Assessment of amniotic fluid volume
- Biophysical profile scoring

Accurate dating of pregnancy

The expected date of delivery is traditionally calculated from the date of the last menstrual period using Naegele's rule (by adding seven days and subtracting three months). This method relies upon accurate history from the patient, a regular menstrual cycle and a patient who was not using hormonal contraceptives at the time of conception. In women with malignant disease, the menstrual cycle may not be reliable secondary to concurrent factors affecting the hypophyseal–pituitary–ovarian axis, e.g., stress, weight loss, radiotherapy and chemotherapy.

In these women, when preterm intervention may be necessary, and perinatal decisions will rely heavily on reliable dates, it is particularly crucial to have ultrasound confirmation of the expected date of delivery. Ultrasound can be used to assess the gestational age of the pregnancy by direct morphometric assessment of the fetus. For any specific measurement, there will be a normal biological variation which is expressed as two standard deviations above and below the mean of the measurement. The rate of fetal growth is exponential at conception and thereafter progressively slower with increasing gestational age. Since the biological variation of the growth indices is inversely proportional to the rate of growth, the earlier the ultrasound is performed in pregnancy, the greater its accuracy for gestational age determination.

The only caveat is that the accuracy of dating from any fetal morphometric will depend upon the accuracy of the measurement itself and the effect of inter- and intraobserver error.

The crown–rump length

The crown–rump length (CRL) is measured of an embryo in the long axis view from the crown of the head and the caudal extremity of the torso. The errors associated with measurement include foreshortening, so the longest axis of the fetus must be used. It is inaccurate if used after 12 weeks' gestation. Within their limits, the estimated error is quoted as ± 3.5 days[20].

Biparietal diameter (BPD)

The biparietal diameter can be measured after 12 weeks but is reliably used for dating after 14 weeks' gestation. The window between 12 and 14 weeks' gestation between CRL and BPD is less reliable for the assessment of gestational age. If used between 14 and 20 weeks' gestation, the error is estimated to be in the region of $\pm$ 1 week. After 20 weeks' gestation, the estimate of error progressively increased to $\pm$ 3 weeks and is less useful in the estimation of gestational age. The specific errors associated with the BPD measurement include variations in shape of head, e.g., dolicocephalic (reduced BPD) or brachycephalic (increased BPD). In these instances head circumference (HC) can be used to aid interpretation of the BPD. In estimating gestational age, HC has not been found to be more accurate than measurement of BPD[21].

Femur length (FL)

The use of the femur length in gestational age assessment was described by O'Brien and Queenan[22] and then by Hadlock *et al*[23]. The femur length is measured by obtaining a long axis view of the femur, and measuring from the midpoints of the greater trochanter to its distal end. The FL can be used to estimate gestation age from 14 weeks with an accuracy of $\pm$ 1 week before 20 weeks' gestation[23].

Serial growth assessment

Ultrasound measurement of fetal biometry can be used in a serial fashion to look at interval growth and growth velocity. Various normogram curves of expected growth have been described which are derived by plotting 5th, 50th and 95th centiles each for morphometric characteristic; these allow restriction of observed fetal growth with that of expected growth. Intrauterine growth restriction is generally defined as a birth-weight below the 10th centile for gestational age. Within this heterogeneous group, there will be fetuses realizing their full growth potential at the lowest end of the normal range as well as "growth-restriction" fetuses. In addition, it must be recognized that some fetuses above the 10th centile may be growth retarded, e.g. falling from the 8th to the 20th centile but will be missed by this definition. Growth velocity can be assessed with serial measurement of fetal biometry and will reveal fetuses in whom growth slows down or fetuses in whom there is real growth retardation whether or not they fall below the 10th centile for estimated fetal weight. In general, this is a much more useful approach to the assessment of intrauterine fetal growth retardation. In women with high-risk pregnancies, e.g., mothers in whom there may be systemic complications of malignancy such as anemia and cachexia, there would be an increased likelihood of compromised fetal growth, and serial ultrasounds at 2–4 week intervals would be advisable to assess fetal growth in the third trimester.

Ultrasound parameters of fetal growth

• Biparietal diameter • Femur length	Assess linear growth. Included in Hadlock formula for estimated fetal weight[24].
• Estimated fetal weight	Different methods described using different parameters: FAC: Campbell & Wilkin 1975[25]. FAC & BPD: Shepard *et al* 1983[26]. FAC, BPD & FL Hadlock *et al* 1985[24].

Asymmetry between the growth of fetal head and abdominal circumference is of importance, since it reflects the "head sparing" effect by which the compromised fetus continues to grow its head but fails to lay down glycogen in the liver, hence a discrepancy between head size and abdominal circumference evolves. This type of growth retardation is called "asymmetric IUGR" and can be distinguished from the symmetrical variety, the former in general terms reflecting placental insufficiency, the latter being more commonly associated with congenital infections and chromosomal abnormality. The appropriate management of a growth-retarded fetus will depend upon its etiology, ranging from the conservative management of an appropriately grown small baby to active intervention and early delivery of a growth-retarded baby with placental insufficiency; and the avoidance of inappropriate intervention in a symmetrically small baby with chromosomal or structural abnormalities.

Assessment of the placenta

The ultrasound is used routinely to assess placental site. The ultrasound assessment of placental architecture to identify "mature" placentas has been described[27], and a grading system devised.

The potential application of placental grading in monitoring the fetus has been studied, although not in great depth. Although placental grade has not been associated with intrauterine growth retardation[28], it has been shown to be predictive of unexplained stillbirth in a low-risk population in a single prospective trial[29].

Although the placental grade is often reported on ultrasound when extreme placental maturity is identified, currently, it is not used clinically in decision-making regarding perinatal management. More work to clarify the clinical role of placental grade is needed, but it is likely that it will be applicable to the screening of a low-risk population rather than the monitoring of an identified high-risk population.

The fetal biophysical profile

In North America particularly, the biophysical profile score has gained huge popularity and widespread use despite a paucity of evidence from randomized controlled trails regarding its benefit on perinatal outcome[30].

In "high-risk" pregnancies it is generally performed twice weekly and can be used from 26–28 weeks' gestation depending upon the clinical situation and whether one would consider acting on the result. It utilizes real time ultrasound to access the fetus over 30 minutes in its intrauterine environment. Fetal breathing, fetal movement, fetal tone and amniotic fluid volume are all assessed and scored as either 2 or zero according to their presence or absence (see Table 5.1).

The biophysical activities of movement and breathing reflect the fetal central nervous system (CNS) function and exhibit cyclical rhythmicity. Two patterns of sleep are recognized, that of quiet sleep and that of active (rapid eye movement sleep). Fetal state will affect breathing, movement and fetal heart rate accelerations all of which are diminished or absent during quiet sleep. This physiological state must be distinguished from the reduced fetal activity observed in response to various stimuli such as hypoxemia, which is thought to represent the fetus's attempt to conserve energy. Suppression of fetal activity is also associated with smoking, alcohol, narcotics, tranquilizers and maternal hypoglycemia.

Whilst fetal biophysical parameters reflect the current fetal condition, and will thus change acutely, the amniotic fluid volume reflects long-term placental function. Reduced amniotic fluid can be associated with poor placental blood flow and chronic hypoxemia (in the absence of a fetal structural abnormality) which lead to reduced blood flow to the fetal kidneys.

By combining the five features of the biophysical profile (BPP) score, it

Table 5.1. *Technique of biophysical profile scoring*

Biophysical variable	Normal (score = 2)	Abnormal (score = 0)
Fetal breathing movements	At least one episode of > 30 seconds duration in 30 minutes' observation	Absent or no episode of ≥ 30 seconds duration in 30 minutes
Gross body movement	At least three discrete body/limb movements in 30 minutes (episodes of active continuous movement considered a single movement)	Up to two episodes of body/limb movements in 30 minutes
Fetal tone	At least one episode of active extension with return to flexion of fetal limb(s) or trunk; opening and closing of hand considered normal tone	Either slow extension with return to partial flexion or movement of limb in full extension or absent fetal movement
Reactive fetal heart rate	At least two episodes of acceleration of ≥ 15 bpm and 15 seconds duration associated with fetal movement in 30 minutes	Fewer than two accelerations or acceleration < 15 bpm in 30 minutes
Qualitative amniotic fluid volume	At least one pocket of amniotic fluid measuring 2 cm in two perpendicular planes	Either no amniotic fluid pockets or a pocket < 2 cm in two perpendicular planes

Adapted from Manning *et al*[33] with permission.

has been possible to reduce false positive test results to as low as 20%. The false negative rate for the BPP is low, i.e., these babies with compromise who had a normal test result, ranging from 6.9/1000 with a normal amniotic fluic volume to 12.8/1000 in fetuses with a reactive NST[31].

The clinical action recommended by Manning in response to BPP scores is presented in Table 5.2[32,33]. However, it is important to individualize care, and to look not just at a BPP *score* but to assess the biophysical findings in the context of the pregnancy as a whole, particularly in situations where the maternal health is poor. In principle, the BPP attempts to examine the fetus as a patient within a patient, and may provide useful information to the clinician coordinating the care of mother and fetus.

Table 5.2. *Management based on biophysical profile*

Score	Interpretation	Management
10	Normal infant; low risk of chronic asphyxia	Repeat testing at weekly intervals; repeat twice weekly in diabetic patients and patients at $\geq$ 42 weeks' gestation
8	Normal infant; low risk of chronic asphyxia	Repeat testing at weekly intervals; repeat testing twice weekly in diabetics and patients at $\geq$ 42 weeks' gestation; oligohydramnios is an indication for delivery
6	Suspect chronic asphyxia	If $\geq$ 36 weeks' gestation and conditions are favorable, deliver; if at $<$ 36 weeks and L/S $<$ 2.0, repeat test in 4–6 hours; deliver if oligohydramnios is present
4	Suspect chronic asphyxia	If $\geq$ 32 weeks' gestation deliver; if $<$ 32 weeks, repeat score
0–2	Strongly suspect chronic asphyxia	Extend testing time to 120 minutes; if persistent score $\geq$ 4, deliver, regardless of gestational age

Adapted from Manning *et al*[32,33] with permission.

Doppler ultrasound

Doppler ultrasound is used to assess uteroplacental blood flows in pregnancy. Unlike most new antenatal tests of fetal well-being, it has been subjected to fairly rigorous prospective evaluation prior to its widespread adaption into a clinical practice. Although all the hopes for the clinical application have not been fully realized, its role in the antenatal care of the high risk patient in conjunction with other modes of assessment of fetal welfare is now recognized.

Doppler systems are available for clinical use in two main forms, continuous-wave and pulsed Doppler; the former relies upon the identification of familiar flow velocity waveform for the vessel being investigated, pulsed "duplex" Doppler systems enable visualization of a specific vessel on which Doppler blood flow studies are performed.

Both fetal and maternal vessels can be studied. In the fetus, Doppler studies of the umbilical artery have the greatest clinical application, although it is possible to Doppler most fetal vessels with a duplex system. The maternal uterine arteries have been studied to assess the maternal blood supply to the placental bed.

Various indices have been devised to quantify the flow velocity waveforms produced whilst remaining independent of the angle of insonance (the angle of insonance is the angle between the Doppler beam and the vessel insonated and *should* ideally be below 30 degrees). The systolic/diastolic ratio (S/D ratio or A/B ratio) is the ratio of the peak systolic(S) to peak diastolic(D) blood flow. The ratio is diminished by large diastolic blood flow, thus high ratios reflect diminished diastolic blood flow.

The pulsating index (PI) is derived from the peak systolic blood flow and then divided by the mean of the velocity waveform profile (S–D/mean). The resistance index (RI) in calculated from S–D/S. Unlike the S/D ratio, the PI and RI can both be used when there is absent or reversed diastolic blood flow.

Meta-analysis of the trials of the use of Doppler ultrasound in pregnancy[34], show a significant reduction in perinatal mortality rate (of 35%) amounted with the use of Doppler ultrasound of the umbilical artery in pregnancy. These findings support the use of umbilical artery ultrasound in the management of high-risk pregnancies. Uteroplacental insufficiency is the underlying pathology in the perinatal deaths avoided using Doppler.

References

1. Sadovsky E, Yaffe H: Daily fetal movement recording and fetal prognosis. *Obstet Gynecol* 1973; 41: 845–50.
2. Sadovsky E, Yaffe H, Polishuk WZ: Fetal movement monitoring in normal and pathologic pregnancy. *Int J Gynaecol Obstet* 1974; 12: 75.
3. Sadovsky E, Polishuk WZ: Fetal movements *in utero*: review. *Obstet Gynecol* 1977; 50: 49–55.
4. Pearson JF, Weaver JB: Fetal activity and fetal wellbeing: an evaluation. *Br Med J* 1976; 1: 1305–7.
5. Neldam S: Fetal movements as an indicator of fetal wellbeing. *Lancet* 1980; i: 1222–4.
6. Patrick J, Carmichael L, Chess L, Staples C: Acceleration of the human fetal heart rate at 38 to 40 weeks' gestational age. *Am J Obstet Gynecol* 1984; 148: 35–41.
7. Grant A, Elbourne D, Valentin L, Alexander S: Routine fetal movements counting and risk of antepartum rate death in normally formed singletons. *Lancet* 1989; ii: 345.
8. Sadovsky E, Ohel G, Havazeleth H: The definition and the significance of decreased fetal movements. *Acta Obstet Gynecol Scand* 1983; 62: 409.
9. Natale R, Clewlow F, Dawes G: Measurement of fetal forelimb movements in the lamb *in utero*. *Am J Obstet Gynecol* 1981; 142: 545.
10. Margulis E, Binder D, Cohen A: The effect of propranolol on the nonstress test. *Am J Obstet Gynecol* 1984; 148: 340.
11. Keegan K, Paul R, Broussard P, McCart D, Smith MA: Antepartum fetal heart rate testing. III. The effect of phenobarbital on the nonstress test. *Am J Obstet Gynecol* 1979; 133: 579.
12. Phelan J: Diminished fetal reactivity with smoking. *Am J Obstet Gynecol* 1980; 136: 230.

13. Lavery J: Nonstress fetal heart rate testing. *Clin Obstet Gynecol* 1982; 25: 689.
14. Keegan K, Paul R, Broussard P, McCart D, Smith MA: Antepartum fetal heart rate testing. V. The nonstress test – an outpatient approach. *Am J Obstet Gynecol* 1980; 136: 81.
15. Meis P, Ureda J, Swain M: Variable decelerations during non-stress tests (NST): a sign of fetal compromise? Society of Perinatal Obstetricians, Fourth Annual Meeting, San Antonio, TX, 1984.
16. Barrett J, Salyer S, Boehm F: The nonstress test: an evaluation of 1000 patients. *Am J Obstet Gynecol* 1981; 141: 153.
17. Miller JM Jr, Horger EO III: Antepartum heart rate testing in diabetic pregnancy. *J Reprod Med* 1985; 30: 515.
18. Gabbe SG, Mestman JH, Freeman RK, Goebelsmann UT, Lowensohn RI, Nochimsom D, Cetrulo C, Quilligan EJ: Management and outcome of diabetes mellitus, class B-R. *Am J Obstet Gynecol* 1977; 129: 723.
19. Ewigman BG, Crane JP, Frigoletto FD, LeFevre ML, Bain RP, McNellis Dj, and the RADIUS Study Group: Effect of prenatal ultrasound screening on perinatal outcome. *N Engl J Med* 1993; 329: 821–7.
20. Robinson H: Sonar measurements of fetal crown–rump lengths as a means of assessing fetal maturity in early pregnancy. *Br Med J* 1973; 4: 28.
21. Hadlock FP, Deter RL, Harrest RB *et al*: Fetal bipariental diameter: rational choice of plane of section for sonographic measurement. *AM J Roentgentol* 1982; 138: 871–4.
22. O'Brien GD, Queenan JT: Growth of the ultrasound femur length during normal pregnancy. *Am J Obst Gynecol* 1981; 141: 833.
23. Hadlock FP, Harrist RB, Deter RL *et al*: Ultrasonically measured fetal femur length as a predictor of menstrual age. *Am J Roentgentol* 1982; 138: 875.
24. Hadlock F, Harrist RB, Deter RL *et al*: Estimation of fetal weight by head, body and femur measurements: a prospective study. *Am J Obst Gynecol* 1985; 151: 333.
25. Campbell S, Wilkin D: Ultrasonic measurement of the fetal abdominal circumference in the estimation of fetal weight. *Br J Obst Gynaecol* 1995; 83: 689.
26. Shepard MJ, Richards VA, Benkowitz RL *et al*: An evaluation of two equations for predicting fetal weight by ultrasound. *Am J Obst Gynecol* 1983; 1432: 47.
27. Grannum PAT, Berkowitz RL, Hobbins JC *et al*: The ultrasonic changes in the maturing placenta and the relationship to fetal pulmonic maturity. *Am J Obst Gynecol* 1975; 133: 915.
28. Harman CR: Ultrasound placental grading: relationship to fetal age, birth weight and birth weight percentile. *Proc Soc Obst Gynecol Canada, Toronto*, 1984.
29. Proud J, Grant AM: Third trimester placental grading by ultrasonography as a test of fetal wellbeing. *Br Med J* 1987; 294: 1641–7.
30. Neilson JP, Alfirevic Z: Biophysical profile for antepartum fetal assessment. In *Pregnancy and Childbirth Module* (Enkin MW, Keirse MJNC, Renfrew MJ, Neilson JP, eds.), *Cochrane Database of Systematic Reviews*: Review no. 07432, 12 May 1994. Published through "Cochrane Updates on Disc", Oxford: Update Software, 1994, Disc Issue 1.
31. Manning F, Platt L, Sipos L: Antepartum fetal evaluation: development of a fetal biophysical profile, *Am J Obstet Gynecol* 1980; 136: 787.
32. Manning FA, Harman CR, Morrison I *et al*: Fetal assessment based on fetal

biophysical profile scoring. *Am J Obstet Gynecol* 1990; 162: 703.
33. Manning F, Baskett T, Morrison I, Lange I: Fetal biophysical profile scoring: a prospective study in 1,184 high-risk patients. *Am J Obstet Gynecol* 1981; 140: 289.
34. Neilson JP: Doppler ultrasound (all trials). In *Pregnancy and Childbirth Module* (Enkin MW, Keirse MJNC, Renfrew MJ, Neilson JP, eds.), *Cochrane Database of Systematic Reviews*: Review No. 07337, 12 May 1994. Published through "Cochrane Updates on Disk", Oxford: Update Software, 1994, Disk Issue 1.

6

The Toronto Study Group: methodological notes

G. KOREN, D. ZEMLICKIS AND M. LISHNER

The study described in this volume is a result of a collaboration between two medical institutions in Toronto: the Princess Margaret Hospital and The Motherisk Program at The Hospital for Sick Children.

Princess Margaret Hospital (PMH) is an oncologic hospital in Toronto serving the province of Ontario. PMH maintains a computerized database of patients' records dating back to 1958, which was used to identify for the study all female patients who had cancer and pregnancy in their diagnosis from 1958 to 1987.

Based on the assumption that cancer would be present for some time before it could be diagnosed, the time frame for inclusion for this analysis selected women who were pregnant within nine months prior or three months after first treatment of their cancer. Nine months were chosen to reflect the normal gestational period and three months to arbitrarily create a time frame of one year (Fig. 6.1).

Since the date of diagnosis was often not recorded in the PMH database, we used the date of first treatment as a reference date, assuming that there would be a minimal delay from the time of diagnosis to treatment (surgical, radiological and/or medical). Extreme cases included in our study were therefore women who delivered nine months before their first treatment and women who conceived three months after the last day of their first treatment.

Potential cases identified by the computer were screened further by examining their charts to confirm that pregnancy and cancer occurred according to the time frame defined above, and to reject any patients who had an ectopic pregnancy.

To study the potential effects of pregnancy on women's survival, we matched women having specific cancers (breast, Hodgkin's and cervix) to nonpregnant women with the same tumor. For each case, an attempt was

                                                     G. Koren, D. Zemlickis and M. Lishner

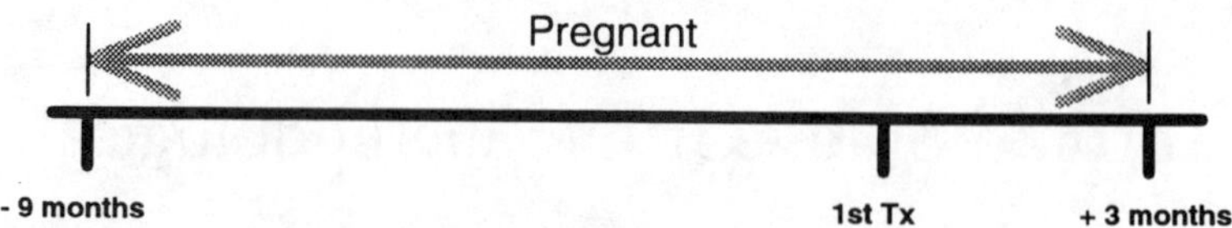

Fig. 6.1   Timeline for selection of cases.

made to identify three matching controls in the PMH database. Criteria for matching are detailed separately for each of the tumors.

For pregnancies that continued to term or resulted in stillbirth, birth records were requested from the delivering hospital. For live births, sex and birthweight of the infant were recorded, as well as gestational age at delivery, type of delivery, Apgar scores, fetal complications, and congenital anomalies. In the case of cesarean section, the reason for choosing this method was recorded. For intrauterine death, the date of diagnosis of the stillbirth and autopsy results were collected.

The Motherisk Program is an antenatal information and consultation service for women and their families and for health professionals regarding exposure to drugs, chemicals, radiation or infections during pregnancy and lactation. Following the expected rate of confinement a follow-up procedure allows detailed description of pregnancy outcome (see Chapter 7).

For the purpose of this study, fetal outcome after specific cancers was compared to that of babies born to women attending the Motherisk Clinic during the first trimester following exposures to drugs, chemicals or radiation during pregnancy. For this analysis, each mother with a specific cancer who had a live birth was matched to a mother of a similar age who was exposed to nonteratogenic drugs or chemicals.

To detect whether any differences in mean birth weight between cases and the Motherisk control group were due to differences in gestational age (e.g., due to decision to induce early labor or perform elective cesarean section) or due to intrauterine growth restriction, birth weight percentile was calculated for the specific gestational age. In addition, analysis of covariance was applied to separate the effect of cancer and gestational age on birth weight.

Cause-specific survival curves were produced using the Kaplan–Meier estimate[1]. For the purposes of this study, cause-specific survival is defined as mortality due to the disease under investigation. Any death caused by other than the disease under investigation was censored. The Mantel–Haenszel log rank test was employed to examine differences between survival curves[2].

A Chi-square test was utilized to compare the distribution of stage upon diagnosis between pregnant cases and nonpregnant controls having the same disease during the reproductive age registered in the PMH data base and to verify that the criteria for matching were similar in cases and controls. The Bonferoni method was used to adjust for multiple comparisons. Fisher's exact test was used to compare proportions.

Fetal outcome values between the study and control groups were compared using a two-sided Student's t-test for independent samples and the Chi-square test whenever appropriate.

The odds ratio was used to estimate the relative risk of a pregnant woman with a specific cancer to have a stillbirth compared to pregnant women without cancer having a stillbirth in the province of Ontario. The observed number of stillbirths was assumed to follow a Poisson distribution. Statistical analysis was performed with the aids of SAS version 5.1 and Minitab release 6.1.1.

Additional analyses are described in the different chapters, as appropriate.

The Appendix displays the forms used for the collection of the data.

CANCER AND PREGNANCY

Note: Please circle appropriate codes   Page 1

1. Patient's name:

2. T No.

_ _ _ _ _ _ _ _ _

3. Age at Dx

_ _ yrs
X X N.S.

4. Birthplace

__________ town/city
__________ province
__________ country

5. Race

White	1
Black	2
Oriental	3
Malayan	4
Indian	6
Other	6
state: ______	

6. Date of cancer Dx.

D̄ D̄ M̄ M̄Ȳ Ȳ
XXXXX N.S.

7. Date of Conception

D̄ D̄ M̄ M̄Ȳ Ȳ
XXXXX N.S.

N.S.   X

8. Date of PMH Reg.

D̄ D̄ M̄ M̄Ȳ Ȳ
XXXXX N.S.

11. Primary Tumour

T1	1
T2	2
T3	3
T4	4
TX	X
N.A.	A

9. Type of Cancer

Breast	1	Melanoma	6
Ovary	2	Hodgkin's	7
Cervix	3	Non-H. Lymph	8
GI Tract	4	Other	9
Leukemia	5	state: ______	
N.S.	X		

10. Stage at Dx

Stage I	1
Stage II	2
Stage III	3
Stage IV	4
N.S.	X
N.A.	A

12. Reg. Lymph Nodes

N0	0	N3	3
N1	1	NX	X
N2	2	N.A.	A

13. Mets. at Dx

Yes	1
No	2
N.S.	X
N.A.	A

14. Site of Mets.

____

N.S.	X
N.A.	A

15. Pathology specific type

Carcinoma ______	1
Lymphoma ______	2
Leukemia ______	3
Sarcoma ______	4
Other ______	5
N.S. ______	X

16. Grade

Well Diff.	1
Mod. Diff.	2
Poorly Diff.	3
N.S.	X

20. Timing of Cancer and Preg.

Preg. Before Rx Began	1
Preg. during RX	2
Preg. after Rx ended	3
N.S.	X

17. First Rx

____

Surgery	1
Radn.	2
Chemo.	3
Other	4
state: ___	
N.S.	X

18. Date of 1st Rx

D̄ D̄ M̄ M̄Ȳ Ȳ
XXXXX N.S.

19. Was Rx Delayed due to Pregnancy?

Yes	1
No	2
N.S.	X
N.A.	A

21. Type of Surg.

____

N.S.	X
N.A.	A

22. Gestat. Age

_ _ _ mos
(+/-)
XXX N.S.

CANCER AND PREGNANCY

Radn./Chemo/Other Drugs
Page 2

23. Total Dose	24. Tumour Dose	25. No. of Fract.	26. Days	27. Target
_ _ _ _ _ rads XXXX N.S. AAAA N.A.	_ _ _ _ rads XXXX N.S. AAAA N.A.	_ _ XX N.S. AA N.A.	_ _ X N.S. A N.A.	_ _ _ _ _ X N.S. A N.A.

28. Shielding	29. Gest. Age

To   Yes   1
Baby   No   2
          N.S.   X
          N.A.   A
	_ _ _ _ _ mos
	(+/-)
	XXX N.S.
	AAA N.A.

30. Chemotherapy Drug   31. Dose   32. Route   33. No. of Courses   34. Gest. Age

35. Other Drug   36. Indication   37. Dose   38. Route   39. No. of Courses   40. Gest.

41. Date of Death/LFU	42. Survival Status	43. Disease Status		
D̄ D̄ M̄ M̄ Ȳ Ȳ XXXXXX N.S.	Alive 0 Dead 1 N.S. X	**If Alive**		**If Dead**

42. Survival Status

Alive   0
Dead   1
N.S.   X

44. Autopsy

Yes   1
No   2
N.S.   X
N.A.   A

43. Disease Status

If Alive		If Dead	
No Disease	1	Of Local Dis.	6
Local Dis.	2	Of Regional Dis.	7
Regional Dis.	3	Of Distant Dis.	8
Distant Dis.	4	Other Cause,	
Dis. Status		With Disease	9
Unknown	5	Other Cause,	
		No Disease	10
		Cause Unknown	11
		Not Known if Alive or Dead	12

CANCER AND PREGNANCY

Outcome of Pregnancy   Page 3

45. Miscarriage

Yes   1
No   2
N.S.   X

46. Date of Misc.

D D M M Y Y
XXXXXX N.S.
AAAAAA N.A.

47. Gest. Age at Misc.

_ _ _ _ mos
XX   N.S.
AA   N.A.

48. Abortion

Yes   1
No   2
N.S.   X

49. Date of Abortion

D D M M Y Y
XXXXXX N.S.
AAAAAA N.A.

50. Gest. Age at Abort.

_ _ _ _ mos
XX   N.S.
AA   N.A.

51. Method

Suction and Curretage   1
Hypertonic Saline   2
Other ___________   3
N.S.   X

52. Reason

Related to Cancer Dx   1
specify: ___________
Not Related to Cancer DX   2
specify: ___________
N.S. X   N.A. A

53. Complic. of Preg.

____
____
N.S. X N.A. A

54. Date of Complic.

D D M M Y Y
XXXXXX N.S.
AAAAAA N.A.

55. Complicat. of Preg.

____
N.S. X N.A. A

56. Date

D D M M Y Y
XXXXXX N.S.
AAAAAA N.A.

57. Sex of Infant

Male   1
Female   2
N.A.   A
N.S.   X

58. Gest. Age at Deliv.

_ _ _ _ mos
XX   N.S.
AA   N.A.

59. Date of Deliv.

D D M M Y Y
XXXXXX N.S.
AAAAAA N.A.

60. Place of Delivery

(Hospital) ___________

(City/Town) ___________

(Country) ___________

X N.S. A.N.

61. Type of Birth

Stillbirth   1
Live Birth   2
N.S.   X
N.A.   A

62. Date of Dx of Stillbirth

D D M M Y Y
XXXXXX N.S.
AAAAAA N.A.

63. Method of Deliv.

Vaginal   1
C/S   2
Forceps/   3
Vacuum
Other ___________ 4   X N.S. A.N.

64. Induction/Accel.

Yes   1
No   2
N.S.   X
N.A.   A

65. Birthweight

_ _ _ _ oz
XXX N.S.
AAA N.A.

68. Method of Gest. Age Determination

Ultrasound   1   N.S.   X
L.M.P.   2   N.A.   A
Blood test   3   Other   4
                  state: ___________

66. Apgar (1)

_ _ _ _
XX   N.S.
AA   N.A.

67. Apgar (5)

_ _ _ _
XX   N.S.
AA   N.A.

69. Malformations

____
X N.S.
A N.A.

70. Complications in Infant

____
X N.S.
A N.A.

CANCER AND PREGNANCY

T No: Page 4

Pt. Name:

Comments

____

____

____

____

____

____

Addresses

Referring MD   Name ____

                      Address ____

                                 ____

                                 ____

Present MD.   Name ____

                      Address ____

                                 ____

                                 ____

                                 ____

                                 ____

                                 ____

Gynecologist   Name ____

                      Address ____

                                 ____

                                 ____

CANCER AND PREGNANCY
NON-PREGNANT CONTROLS

Dr. Koren
Dr. Sutcliffe
Dr. Lishner

Control must not have been pregnant for 15 mos prior to dx of cancer or for 9 months after dx.

Control must be pre-menopausal

1. PATIENT'S NAME ____

2. T NUMBER ____________________________ 3. AGE AT DX __________ YRS

4. MATCHED WITH ____

5. BIRTHPLACE	6. RACE			
______________ town/city	White	1	Malayan	4
______________ province	Black	2	Indian	5
______________ country	Oriental	3	Other State:	
	N.S.	X	______________	

7. DATE OF CANCER DX	8. DATE OF PMH REGISTRATION
______________	______________
DDMMYY	DDMMYY
N.S. X	N.S. X

9. TYPE OF CANCER	
Breast 1 Melanoma 6	
Hodgkin's 7 N.S. X	
Cervix 3	

10. CLINICAL T ____ N ____ M ____	11. PATHOLOGICAL T ____ N ____ M ____
OR STAGE ______	OR STAGE ______

12. SITE OF METS.	13. PATHOLOGY	14. GRADE
______________	Carcinoma ______ 1	Well. Diff. 1
N.S. X	Lymphoma ______ 2	Mod. Diff. 2
N.A. A	Other ______ 3	Poorly D. 3
	N.S. ______ X	Undiff. 4
		N.S. X

15. 1ST TX	16. DATE OF 1ST TX	17. TYPE OF SURGERY
Surgery 1	______________	______________
Radiation 2	DDMMYY	
Chemo 3	N.S. X	N.S X
Other State:		N.A. A
______________		

XRT INFORMATION

XRT FROM ______________ (DDMMYY)	TO ______________ (DDMMYY)

18. TOTAL DOSE	19. NO. OF FRACT.	20. DAYS	21. TARGET
______ rads	___	___	______
XXXX N.S.	XX N.S.	XX	XX N.S.
AAAA N.A.	AA N.A.	AA	AA N.A.

CHEMOTHERAPY INFORMATION

CHEMO FROM ______________ (DDMMYY)	TO ______________ (DDMMYY)

22. CHEMO DRUG	23. DOSE	24. ROUTE	25. NO. OF COURSES

26. DATE OF DEATH/LFU	27. SURVIVAL STATUS	28. AUTOPSY
______ DDMMYY	Alive 1 Dead 2	Yes 1 No 2 N.S. X N.A. A

29. DISEASE STATUS

If Alive		If Dead	
No Disease	1	Of Local Dis.	6
Local Dis.	2	Of Regional Dis.	7
Regional Dis.	3	Of Distant Dis.	8
Distant Dis.	4	Other Cause, With Disease	9
Dis. Status Unknown	5	Other Cause, No Disease	10
		Cause Unknown	11

References

1. Kaplan EL, Meier P: Nonparametric estimation from incomplete observations. *J Am Stat Assoc* 1958; 53: 457–81.
2. Peto R, Pike MS, Armitage P *et al*: Design and analysis of randomized clinical trials requiring prolonged observation of each patient. *Br J Cancer* 1977; 35: 1–39.

7

Motherisk: the process of counselling in reproductive toxicology

G. KOREN AND A. PASTUSZAK

Introduction

Since its inception in 1985, it has become apparent to members of the Motherisk Program that consultations regarding cancer treatment during pregnancy, albeit rare, are amongst the most difficult to handle (Table 7.1). In addition to the insurmountable emotional and clinical difficulties, the data to base rational risk–benefit analysis were sparse or missing. This was the driving force for the initiation of the studies that have led to this volume. The present chapter will focus on description of the Motherisk Program, its mandate and operation.

Since the thalidomide tragedy, there has been an increased awareness of the potential for drugs, chemicals, and radiation to interfere with embryogenesis and/or development of the fetus. Traditionally, women have relied on their physicians and on the media (books, magazines, and television) for answers regarding concerns about drug exposure during pregnancy. Within the past couple of years, a specialized form of information service (the teratogen information service) has appeared in a number of cities in the United States and Canada. The main function of a teratogen information service is to provide information (in all cases) and consultation (in a few cases) to health professionals and/or the general public who have concerns with respect to drug, chemical, and radiation exposure during pregnancy, to determine any potential risk to the pregnant patient and/or to her unborn child. This chapter describes the Motherisk Program located at the Hospital for Sick Children in Toronto, Ontario, Canada, with special emphasis on its day-to-day operation. The description includes the program mandate, protocols for both the telephone information and clinic consultation components, offspring follow-up, technical support, staffing, and direction for the future.

Table 7.1. *Clinic consultations regarding drugs used in the treatment of cancer (Motherisk 1985–1991)*

Drug	Number of cases
Adriamycin	2
Azathioprine	2
Bleomycin	2
Busulfan	1
Cyclophosphamide	4
Danazol	12
Interferon	4
Laetril	2
Methocarbomol	5
Methotrexate	6
Prednisone	82[*]
Procarbazine	2
Vinblastine	1
Vincristine	5

[*]Most patients were not treated for cancer.

Inception

Before I knew I was pregnant, I had a chest X-ray. Will this harm my baby?
I have a patient who requires therapy for UTI. Can I prescribe cephalexin?
I have Crohn's disease. What are the risks to me and my baby should I become pregnant?

Can I have my hair permed during pregnancy?

These are the types of questions members of the Division of Pharmacology and Toxicology at the Hospital for Sick Children have received in the past few years, perhaps owing to increasing awareness on the part of physicians and their patients (pregnant or not) that various xenobiotics have the potential to cross the placenta and possibly to interfere with fetal development. It became apparent that a protocol should be developed to adequately assess the risk or lack of risk, and the concept of the Motherisk Program ensued. The program began operation in September 1985, first as a consultation service in a clinic setting; it has since expanded to include a telephone information service.

Mandate

The goal of Motherisk is twofold:
1. to provide an authoritative information and consultation service to assist the pregnant patient and/or her physician in understanding fetal

risk(s) that may be associated with drug, chemical, and radiation exposure(s) during pregnancy;
2. to develop and maintain active educational and research programs in the area of reproductive and developmental toxicology at the undergraduate, graduate, and postgraduate levels.

Telephone information service

The telephone information service of the Motherisk Program is available to health professionals and to the general public. Incoming calls are received by the information specialist, who at the time of the call decides whether the caller should be referred for a clinic appointment or to the physician on call, or whether the query is such that the information specialist may answer the call satisfactorily. The following criteria are used to determine whether the caller should be referred to clinic:

1. chronic illness (e.g., epilepsy, cancer systemic lupus erythematosus, Crohn's disease);
2. substance abuse (e.g., cocaine, alcohol, heroin);
3. known or suspected teratogen (e.g., phenytoin, antineoplastics);
4. pregnancy complicated by psychosocial problems;
5. physician referral to clinic;
6. multiple exposures;
7. any woman who may not fit into the categories above but requests a clinic visit (i.e., high level of maternal anxiety).

Questions about uncomplicated single or multiple exposures (e.g., most antibiotics and analgesics) are usually answered over the telephone by the information specialist. Physicians who wish to consult with respect to various drug protocols are referred to the physician on call.

In all these queries it is essential to determine potential risk factors involving the patient, regardless of whether she is seen in the clinic or evaluated over the telephone. Not only is proper identification of the drug/chemical involved essential but it is also very important to define the dose, time of exposure in gestation, toxicological events, underlying disease states, and other concomitant drug therapy. It is not uncommon for callers, usually physicians, to question the safety of a medication before they prescribe it. In the cases of questionable safety or lack of information, other modes of treatment may be suggested. In addition to the foregoing inquiries relating to the exposure in question, it is necessary to inquire about past medical history, since not infrequently what seems to be unimportant to the caller may influence the evaluation of risk. For example, a caller who questions paternal marijuana use and the potential effect on her unborn child may, upon questioning, reveal that she has epilepsy and is being treated with phenytoin. In this case, the caller should be provided with information regarding the potential risks with respect to phenytoin treatment and epilepsy *per se*, in addition to the paternal exposure to marijuana.

Callers such as the woman in the example above, whose risk is deemed to be above the baseline for malformations, are usually referred to the clinic for further consultation. When there is no apparent increase above the baseline, the caller is provided with information and an explanation of baseline risk. It is necessary to ensure that each caller understands the concept of the general population risk for having a child with a malformation and that her exposure does not increase this risk.

The Motherisk Telephone Call Report Form is completed for all calls received. All calls are entered daily into a separate data base from the clinic consults and daily summary sheets are retained for quick reference and follow-up. Monthly summary sheets are used both for statistical purposes and for quality assurance.

Presently, the Motherisk Program receives approximately 2000 telephone queries per month, an increase of sixfold since the inception of the telephone component. Long-distance calls comprise approximately 18% of the monthly total, with most calls originating outside the Toronto area code. Callers question, on average, 1.46 exposures. Of these calls, 2–5% are scheduled for clinical appointments. Of the calls, 25% come from health professionals, and the majority (> 85%) are from physicians. The remainder are made up of pharmacists and public health nurses. The most common calls question the safety of various prescription medications (51%), followed by over-the-counter medications (19%), chemicals (15%), recreational substances (7%), radiation (6%), and infections (3%).

Telephone follow-up

Follow-up of pregnancy outcome is performed in all cases in which women are consulted in the clinic. In addition, the following selected cases (usually those in which information was provided over the telephone) are contacted.

Motherisk: Telephone Call Report Form   Date_________________ Time

Patient Name_________________ Phone #_________ Caller_________
                                                Address_________

Parity________ Age_____ Referral_________________ Phone#_________

PREGNANT   **NOT PREG.**   Phone Call Returned_________
                                                No Answer (time & day)_________
______wks/mos at time of expos. Gen. Info_____ No Answer (time & day)_________
                                                Message left _________
______wks/mos currently   Planning______
                                                HEALTH -
BREASTFEEDING_______   Retro_______   General_________

          Exposure Details   _________

Drug Name   Dose/Duration   Route Indication   Toxicology

1._________________ ______________   _____ __________ ______________

2._________________ ______________   _____ __________ ______________

3._________________ ______________   _____ __________ ______________

4._________________ ______________   _____ __________ ______________

          ADVISED   No increase above baseline 3%_________

Reference(s):   Baseline risk was explained_________
_________________________   Referred for clinic appointment
_________________________   (date/time)_________

Advised:
Other_________
____
____

          BREASTFEEDING   Advised: Re
                                       Breastfeeding_________

Age of Infant_________   _________

Times per day_________   _________
Follow-Up   YES___   _________

             NO___
Date:_________   _________

Comments:_________   Signature of
                                       Respondent_________

Fig. 7.1   Motherisk telephone call report form.

1. All inquiries on drugs and breastfeeding to record any medical complications.
2. Cases not seen in the clinic, yet the knowledge of pregnancy outcome is desirable (such as new drugs about which no information currently exists)

The telephone follow-up is conducted either by the information specialist or by pharmacology–toxicology undergraduate students affiliated with

Motherisk. A more detailed discussion of the follow-up process can be found later in this chapter.

The results of the follow-up of pregnancy outcome are added to the Motherisk data-base and are used to generate new data on the safety of drugs and chemicals in pregnancy. When following women not seen in clinic, a maternal data form is completed in addition to the offspring form to ensure uniformity.

Clinic consultation

Approximately 2–5% of Motherisk callers are referred to the clinic. All patents scheduled are seen by a physician affiliated with Motherisk. Fig. 7.2 shows the maternal data form used during the clinic interview. In addition to the primary exposure data, details on other potential risk factors are recorded. These include obstetrical and past medical history, genetic background, additional exposures other than medications, occupation, and paternal exposures.

Prior to presentation of the known data concerning the exposure in question, the patient is asked to complete the visual analog scale (VAS) illustrated in Fig. 7.3. This visual analog aids the physician in determining the patient's concept of her own risk, thus providing direction for the remainder of the interview. A study conducted by members of Motherisk has shown that women exposed to nonteratogens assign themselves, on average, a risk of one in four for having a child with malformation. It was also shown that these women know the baseline risk in the general population, suggesting that other factors may play a significant role in the patient's interpretation of her own risk.

Following this procedure, the physician presents to the woman the available information on her particular reproductive risk/no risk, with special focus on the teratogenic risk in the general population. Subsequently, the visual analog scale is repeated to aid the physician in determining how well the patient understands the information presented. When using the visual analog, it becomes very obvious, especially in cases in which no increased teratogenic risk exists, if certain aspects need to be clarified.

In a variety of cases, additional tests may be deemed necessary by the counseling physician. These commonly include a level 2 ultrasound to rule out visible malformations, or a referral to our genetic clinic to assess, in depth, the genetic background or to arrange for an amniocentesis (e.g., age-related Down's syndrome or increased risk for neural tube defects with exposure to valproic acid).

MOTHERISK

ANTENATAL CLINIC FOR DRUG/CHEMICAL RISK COUNSELLING

THE DIVISION OF CLINICAL PHARMACOLOGY, HOSPITAL FOR SICK CHILDREN

TORONTO, ONTARIO

MOTHERISK NO.____

DATE OF CONSULTATION:____

HSC NUMBER____

1.   **MATERNAL DATA**

Name: ____ ___________________

Address: ____
____

Phone Number: (Home)____________________   (Work)____________________

Husband's Name & Work Number____

O.H.I.P. #____________________________ Date of Birth _____________________________

Race/Ethnic Background____

Weight (dry/current):____

Physician's name: _____________________________   _____________________________

Address: _____________________________   _____________________________

Phone Number:_____________________________   _____________________________

[   ] Self-Referred   [   ] Referred by her doctor

2.   **OBSTETRICAL HISTORY**

Past Obstetrical History (G-P-Ab):____

____

____

____

Birth Control Methods:____

Duration: ____

Date stopped: ____

Fig. 7.2   Motherisk maternal intake history form.

2

Ovulatory Drugs: ____

LMP:_______________ [ ] Regular Mens. [ ] Irregular Mens.   # of days__________

EDC:____

Current Gestational Date:____

When did she find out she was pregnant?____________________
How? [ ] Blood test   [ ] Urine test   [ ] Ultrasound

3.   PRIMARY EXPOSURE DATA

1 = DRUG, 2 = CHEMICAL, 3 = RADIATION
4 = NOT PREGNANT(PROSPECTIVE), 5 = RETROSPECTIVE
A = ADVERTANT I = INADVERTANT

Exposure type (1-5) (A or I)	Substance	Duration		Dosage	Route
		Beg. Date	Stop Date		

Indication for
Medication:____

____

More Details about Medical Condition:___________________________________

____

____

Figure 7.2   (continued)

3

Toxicology Events:____

____

____

Side Effects of Medication:____

____

Ultrasound Data:____

Ultrasound Results:____

Amniocentesis planned for:_______ ___________Reason___________________________

Additional Exposures:

<u>Substance</u>	<u>Dates</u>	<u>Dosage</u>	<u>Rout</u>	<u>Indication</u>

Ethanol:____

Tobacco:____

Heat:____

Radiation:____

Tea & Coffee:____

Special Diet:____

Drugs of Abuse:____

Occupation:____

Genetic diseases or malformations in the family:____

____

____

Figure 7.2   (continued)

4

Past Medical History:

Heart disease:____

Hypertension:____

Renal disease:____

Diabetes:____

Thyroid disease:____

Epilepsy:____

Cancer:____

General Anaesthesia:____

Other:____

[ ] Married
[ ] Single

4.   **SPOUSE DATA**

Age:____

Occupation:____

Medication:____

Drugs of Abuse:____

Ethanol:____

Tobacco:____

Past Medical History:

____
____
____
____
____

Figure 7.2   (continued)

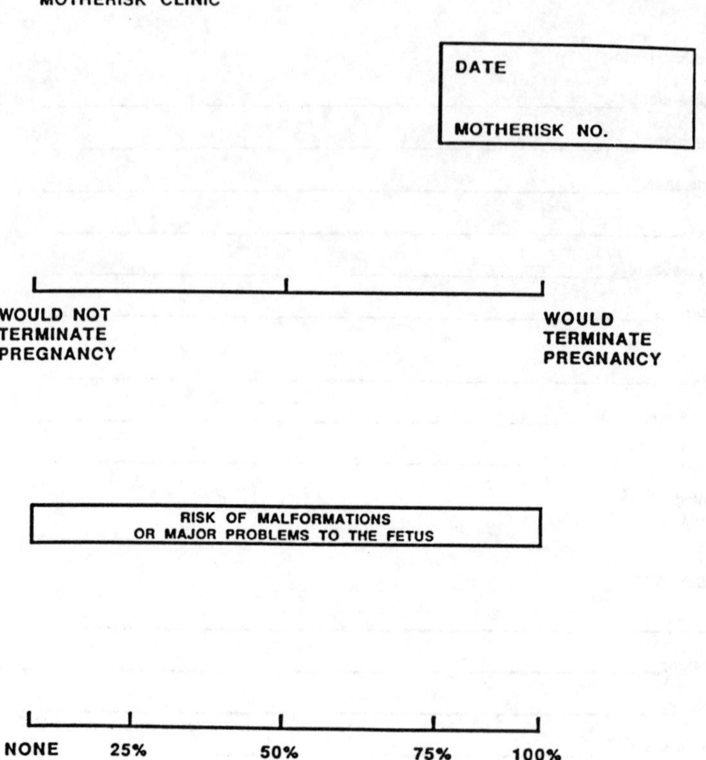

Fig. 7.3   Maternal estimate of risk of malformed offspring.

Following the clinic visit, a letter is sent to the physician(s) caring for the woman during her pregnancy, summarizing the information presented at Motherisk. Upon request, a copy of the letter may also be sent to the patient.

Follow-up of pregnancy outcome

Approximately 12 months following the expected birth of the offspring, all Motherisk patients are contacted for a follow-up interview. Normally, this interview is conducted over the telephone using the Motherisk offspring form. A separate form is subsequently sent to the child's pediatrician to obtain further information. The consent form for release of information, signed during the initial Motherisk interview, is used for this purpose. All data gathered are then entered into the Motherisk data base for analysis.

In specific research cohorts the patient is asked to return to the clinic with her child. The intake form for this visit is identical to the one used for the telephone interview, but in addition, depending on the protocol, the child may be examined by a pediatrician/geneticist.

Technical support

All information regarding patients and their children seen in Motherisk is stored in a data base with built-in levels of security, to limit access to patient information. The hard copy of the patient interview is stored in the Motherisk office. Data base management is the responsibility of the coordinator, though simple data entry may be performed by other health professionals.

The data base program was designed at the Hospital for Sick Children.

In addition to personal computers, the Motherisk office is linked via modem to the mainframe VAX in the hospital for more complex problem solving and for accessing Bibliographic Retrieval Services for MEDLINE searches. The ability to perform these searches in the office rather than contracting them out provides greater flexibility within the program, since the waiting time for the information is decreased.

Staff

The Motherisk staff is drawn from various areas of the health sciences because the evaluation of reproductive risk requires a multidisciplinary approach.

Postdoctoral MD fellows trained at the Division of Pharmacology and Toxicology are on call for at least one week a month. In addition, each of the fellows participates in counseling patients in clinic and in developing new protocols for strategies for the program.

The Motherisk team meets once weekly before clinic to review recent publications, to discuss current cases, and to formulate new protocols from both research and service point of view. The protocols and strategies that ensue from these meetings are stored on a word-processing document that is continuously revised and updated. The information contained therein forms the backbone for the telephone information component as well as the clinic component of Motherisk. In addition, this information is included in all letters dealing with specific exposures.

Information that is used in the consultation process is gathered from a number of sources. The medical information specialist on the team searches current journals for any new information published on drug, chemical, and radiation exposures during pregnancy in either animals or humans. These studies are then analyzed by the team to determine whether the study merits inclusion in our protocols. New textbooks are also searched for relevant information. If a question regarding an uncommon exposure or a new drug is raised, a MEDLINE search is performed to obtain any information that might be available. In the case of new agents, for which no information has yet been published, the manufacturer is contacted for a summary of the voluntary reporting system adhered to, and for premarketing animal studies. In certain cases, experts in a particular field may be called upon to provide insight into a particular exposure. When all the information has been gathered, it is evaluated and submitted for inclusion in protocol and strategy documents for use in future cases.

Educational component

During the academic year, the Motherisk Program involves undergraduate and graduate students from the Department of Pharmacology and Toxicology at the University of Toronto in various projects. This has proven to be an invaluable learning experience for the students, in addition to providing the program with more opportunity to expand research activities. The postgraduate medical fellows in clinical pharmacology participate in the educational program by supervising specific research projects.

Support

The Ministry of Health of Ontario supports the positions of the information specialists as telephone and computer expenses. All other positions are part of the educational curriculum of the involved divisions and departments. Patient consultations are billed through the Ontario Health Insurance Program (OHIP), but physician involvement in telephone information and consultation is not billed. Research protocols compete for extramural support at the appropriate agencies, and the generated funds are dedicated to answer the specific research questions (e.g., cocaine in pregnancy).

Motherisk satellites

Programs similar to Motherisk are located throughout the Province of Ontario, including centers such as Ottawa and Hamilton. Smaller centers located in remote northern parts of Ontario consult Motherisk directly. It is hoped that, by combining the data from the various centers, a strong data base will be created. Such a resource is needed especially for the estimation of teratogenic risk of new compounds for which there is currently no information available.

Summary

The Motherisk Program represents a new clinical approach to the problems of estimating reproductive risk following exposure to drugs, chemicals, and radiation. While the primary goal is to provide a needed service to women and their physicians, a prospective data base enables us to collect information on pregnancy outcome following exposure to agents on which there are no data.

Part II
Specific tumors during pregnancy

8
Maternal and fetal outcome following breast cancer in pregnancy

D. ZEMLICKIS, M. LISHNER, P. DEGENDORFER,
T. PANZARELLA, S. B. SUTCLIFFE AND
G. KOREN

Cancer occurring during pregnancy poses a very difficult challenge to the woman, her family and her physicians, because therapy of her cancer may be detrimental to the unborn baby. Equally difficult, postponement of her therapy may theoretically decrease her chances of survival. Traditionally, cancer during pregnancy was believed to be associated with poor prognosis and an increased risk of harm to the fetus[1-3]. This impression may have led to unnecessary fear on the part of the patient and her physician; conversely, some recent studies have indicated that the pessimistic view is not based on objective data[4-7].

Breast cancer is the most common tumor in women of reproductive age; 3% of breast cancer occurs in pregnancy[8,9]. Because of the relative rareness of breast cancer in pregnancy, there is paucity of information on the effects of pregnancy on the course of breast cancer, and the effect of the disease and its therapy on pregnancy outcome.

Using a large database accumulated for over 30 years in an oncologic hospital in Toronto, we undertook an historical cohort study to assess the effects of pregnancy on the diagnosis and course of breast cancer and the impact of the disease and its treatment on fetal outcome.

Methods

To study the potential effects of pregnancy on women's survival, we matched women having breast cancer in pregnancy to nonpregnant women with the tumor. For each case, an attempt was made to identify three matching controls in the PMH data base according to the following criteria:

(a) The control woman could not have been pregnant within 15 months prior to 9 months after first treatment. A 6-month addition on both sides of the time frame ensured that a pregnancy would have no effect on the cancer and that the cancer would have no effect on a pregnancy.

(b) Controls had the same stage of breast cancer as the cases at diagnosis. The clinical stage was used for both cases and controls when available and pathological when the clinical stage was not recorded (Table 8.1).

(c) Controls were within two years of age of the cases at diagnosis.

(d) Controls were diagnosed and/or had their first treatment within two calendaric years of the matched case. Type of treatment was not explicitly matched; however, strict hospital protocol dictated that patients of the same age, stage, and calendaric year of diagnosis would be given the same treatment. The validity of this assumption was verified in a random sample of 10 pregnant women and 20 controls, which showed identical treatment in 16 (80%) and very similar treatment in the remaining 4 (20%) (minor changes in protocol).

Details of the breast cancer, TNM staging, and date of diagnosis were recorded for the cases and controls. All cases and controls were rated by the TNM system of 1987[10]. Charts with an ambiguous TNM rating were assessed from their pathology reports and clinical workup. Table 8.1 illustrates the staging method.

Dates and types of treatment including whether treatment was delayed due to the pregnancy were also obtained. For obstetrical information, date of conception, gestational age at diagnosis and first treatment, complications in pregnancy, if any, and pregnancy outcome were recorded.

To compare the distribution of disease stages upon diagnosis of breast cancer in pregnancy to that of nonpregnant women of reproductive age ($< = 47$ years) registered in the PMH, the PMH data base was utilized, where 3949 cases had an identifiable stage and an additional 1166 cases were identified as clearly not being stage 4 (either 1, 2, or 3) for the same calendaric years.

Results

There were 118 cases of breast cancer and pregnancy identified in the 30 years analyzed in our study. One woman had two pregnancies, both of which fit in the time frame of the study, resulting in a total of 119 pregnancies in 118 women. The mean age of breast cancer pregnant patients was 32.9 ± 5.1 years upon diagnosis. The median age was 33 years (range 23 to 47). Of the 119 pregnancies, 14 women were diagnosed with breast cancer before conception, 42 during the pregnancy, and 55 women

Table 8.1. *Staging method*

T	N	M	Stage
TO	NO	MO	0
T1, T2, T3	NO	MO	1
T1, T2, T3	N1, N2, N3	MO	2
T4	Any	MO	3
Any	Any	M1	4

Table 8.2. *Types of first treatment*

Type of first treatment	Pregnant women with breast cancer ($n = 118$)
Surgery	22
Radiation	5
Chemotherapy	3
Surgery and radiation	45
Radiation and chemotheraphy	2
Surgery, radiation, and chemotheraphy	21

after delivery or termination of the pregnancy. In eight cases it was not recorded when conception occurred relative to diagnosis.

Out of 118 women, 22 had surgery as first treatment, 5 were irradiated, 3 received chemotherapy, 45 had surgery and radiation, 20 received surgery and chemotherapy, 2 received radiation and chemotherapy, and 21 received all three (Table 8.2). Of the women who were diagnosed prior to, or during, the pregnancy ($n = 56$) and received treatment during the pregnancy ($n = 42$), 24 had surgery, 5 were irradiated, 2 received chemotherapy, 3 had both surgery and chemotherapy, and 8 had both surgery and radiation. Of this group of women, there were 16 therapeutic abortions, 2 miscarriages and 38 live births. Sixteen women chose to delay the recommended treatment until after delivery or termination (two of whom received surgery and delayed chemotherapy). Only five babies were exposed in utero to cancer chemotherapy; three of them during embryogenesis. These three women chose to therapeutically terminate the pregnancy.

There were 269 matched controls identified for 102 cases. Three controls per patient could not always be obtained because the matching criteria were selective enough that the PMH patient database did not always contain three matches per case. For those women who had matched controls, the distribution of types of treatment between cases and controls was not statistically different (p > .75). There were 16 cases that did not have matched controls.

Six patients were diagnosed with breast cancer in the late 1950s or early 1960s and could not be matched because computer records of that time contained ambiguous staging codes. Seven patients had no matches because the patients could not be properly staged, and the remaining three had no matches in the data base. Review of these 16 charts did not reveal any systematic features that would explain why these patients could not be matched.

A Kaplan–Meier plot reveals that survival did not differ statistically between the pregnant and nonpregnant women (p = 0.6, Fig. 8.1). At the time of the study, 52 of the cases had died of breast cancer while the remaining 50 were either alive or died of other causes. In the control group, 129 patients died of breast cancer.

Fig. 8.2 compares the subgroup of patients who were diagnosed with breast cancer prior to conception or during pregnancy ($n = 44$) with their matched controls ($n = 118$), showing virtually identical survival over 15 years (p = 0.5).

For women who were diagnosed with breast cancer during pregnancy and maintained the pregnancy until delivery ($n = 32$), 5 were diagnosed during the first trimester, 11 during the second, and 16 during the third. Fig. 8.3 shows no statistical significant difference in survival between the 3 trimesters (p = 0.8). Fig. 8.4 compares the survival of women who maintained the pregnancy until delivery ($n = 32$) to those who terminated either therapeutically ($n = 9$) or spontaneously ($n = 1$). No statistically significant difference was found (p = 0.5). Women who delayed their treatment until after delivery did not have worse prognosis than their matched controls (11 cases and 28 controls) (p = 0.05). However, because of the small sample sizes in Figs. 8.3 and 8.4 the power is low.

Out of 111 cases, with available staging, 51 (45.9%) had stage 1 disease at diagnosis, 44 (39.6%) stage 2, 6 (5.4%) stage 3, and 10 (9.0%) had stage 4. Their cause-specific survival by stages is shown in Fig. 8.5. A statistically significant difference in survival was found between the stages (p = 0.001).

Through the computerized data base, we identified 3949 women of reproductive age ($< = 47$ yrs), in the same time period (1858–1987), for whom complete staging was available, and an additional 1166 women for whom partial information could confidently rule out stage 4 disease.

Of the 3949 women, 2288 (57.9%) were diagnosed with stage 1 disease, 1293 (32.7%) with stage 2, and 169 (4.3%) with stage 3. There were 199 women diagnosed with stage 4 disease out of 5115 eligible cases (3.9%).

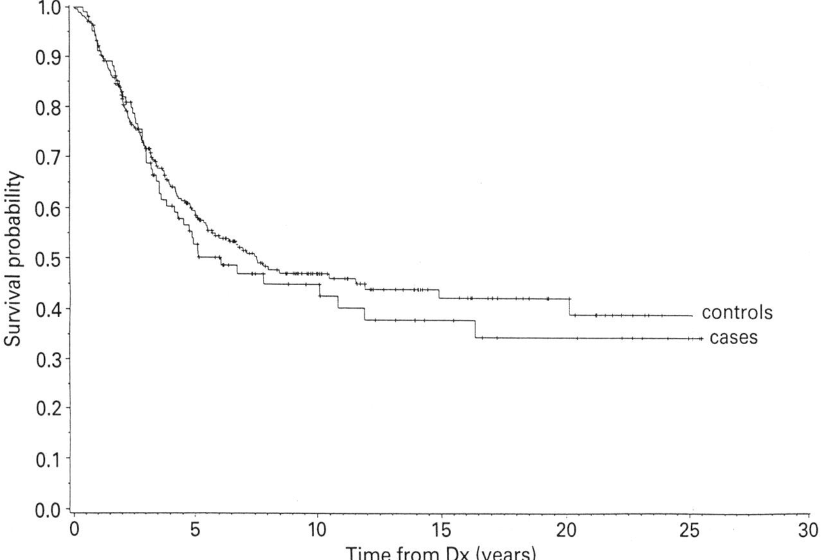

Fig. 8.1   Kaplan–Meier cause-specific survival curve for breast cancer comparing women who were pregnant and had breast cancer ($n = 102$) against matched nonpregnant controls ($n = 269$).

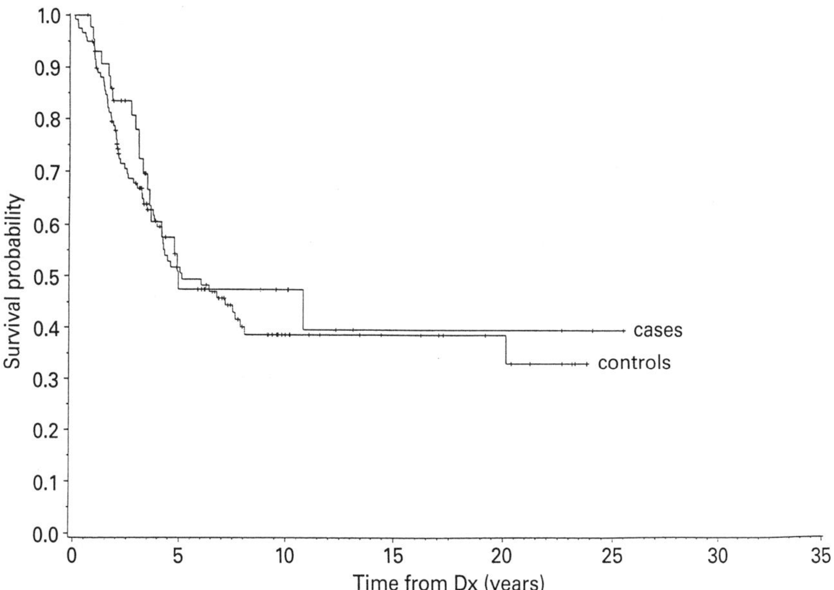

Fig. 8.2   Kaplan–Meier cause-specific survival curve for breast cancer comparing women who were diagnosed before or during pregnancy ($n = 44$) against their nonpregnant matched controls ($n = 118$). p = 0.5.

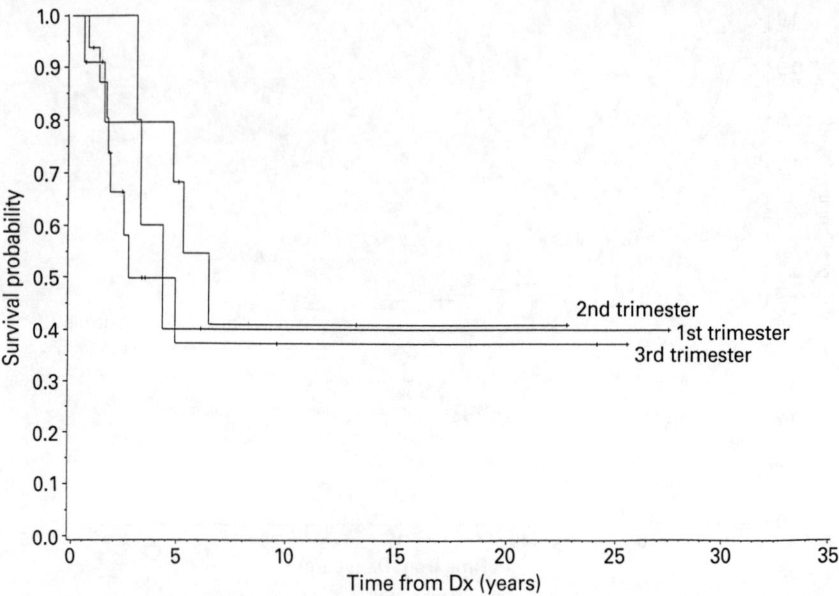

Fig. 8.3   Kaplan–Meier cause-specific survival curve for breast cancer comparing survival for pregnant women diagnosed during first ($n = 5$), second ($n = 11$), and third ($n = 16$) trimester. p = 0.8.

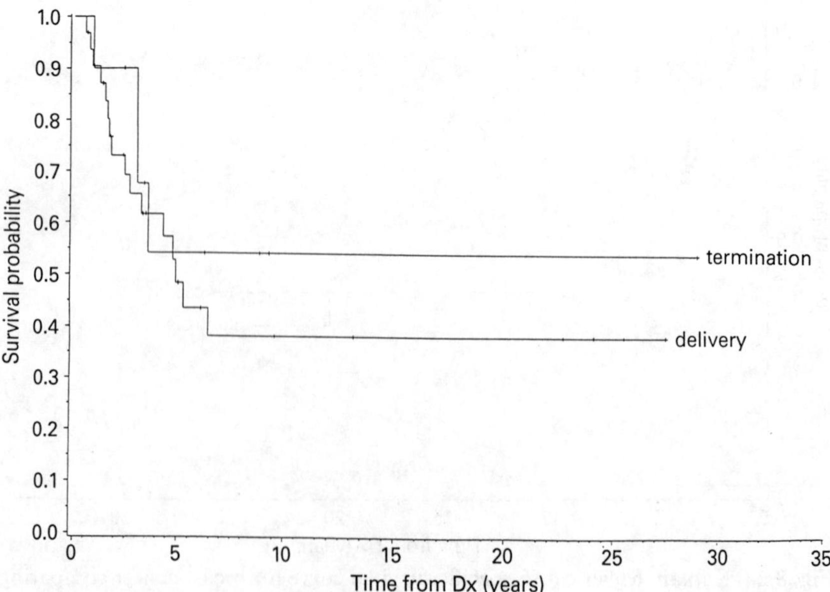

Fig. 8.4   Kaplan–Meier cause-specific survival curve for breast cancer comparing women who delivered ($n = 32$) against those who terminated ($n = 10$). p = 0.5.

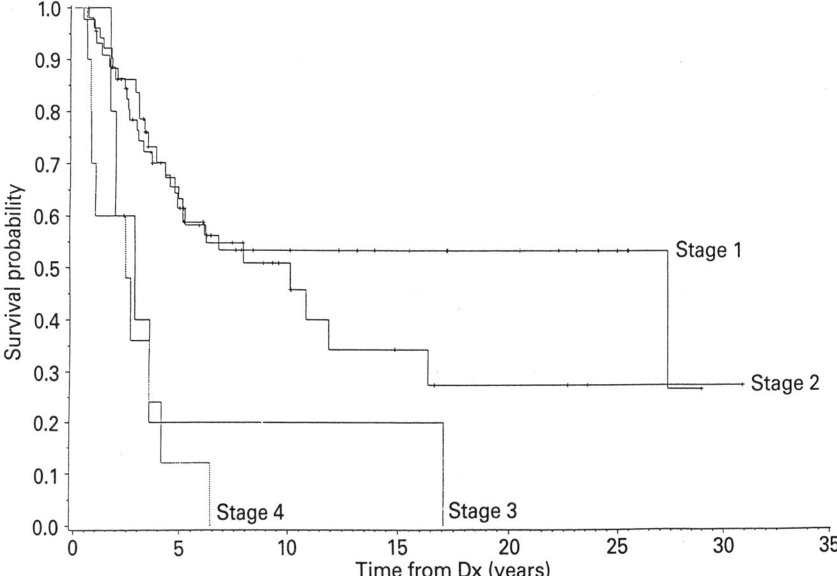

Fig. 8.5 Kaplan–Meier cause-specific survival curve for breast cancer of pregnant women by stage. Stage 1 ($n = 51$), Stage 2 ($n = 44$), Stage 3 ($n = 6$), Stage 4 ($n = 10$). p = 0.001.

This distribution is statistically significantly different from that of the pregnant women ($0.025 < p < 0.05$). When analyzed by individual stage, and adjusted for multiple comparisons (Bonferroni method), a statistically lower number of women diagnosed with stage 1 disease in the pregnant group was found compared with the PMH data base (p = 0.015). Similarly, after adjusting for multiple comparisons, there was a statistically higher proportion of women diagnosed with stage 4 disease in the pregnant group compared to the PMH data base (p = 0.013). The relative risk of having stage 4 disease in pregnancy was 2.5 (95% CI of 1.1 to 5.3).

Fetal outcome

Of the 119 pregnancies, 22 were terminated by therapeutic abortions, 12 by miscarriages, and there were 85 deliveries. Of the 85 deliveries, there were 83 live births and 2 still-births. Of the deliveries 21 were by cesarean section; 18 of these were performed to allow initiation of therapy for breast cancer while the remaining 3 for non cancer-related obstetrical difficulties. We were able to obtain 62 obstetrical records from the delivering hospitals and 1 autopsy report. The remaining delivery records could not be obtained

D. Zemlickis et al.

Table 8.3. *Comparison of fetal outcome in mothers with breast cancer to the matched control group (n = 73)*

	n	Study babies	n	Matched control babies
Mean gestational age	60	38.3 ± 2.4 weeks[a]	73	39.4 ± 1.8 weeks[a]
Number of preterm births (< 37 weeks)	60	16	73	5
Mean birth weight	44	3010 ± 787 g[b]	73	3451 ± 515 g**
Delivery method	57	37 spontaneous 20 cesarean	73	59 spontaneous 14 cesarean
Malformations	73	None	73	None

[a] $p = 0.006$.
[b] $p = 0.002$.
[c] Plus–minus values are means $\pm$ SD.

because some PMH charts did not indicate the delivering hospital or the delivering hospital had destroyed old birth records. In some cases the delivering hospital refused to release confidential documents due to strict hospital guidelines. A summary of the available information regarding fetal outcome is presented in Table 8.3.

There was a statistically lower mean birth weight for babies of mothers with breast cancer when compared to their matched controls ($p = 0.002$). Similarly, they had a statistically shorter mean gestational age ($p = 0.006$) due to a significantly higher proportion of preterm deliveries.

To assess whether the lower birth weight in babies of cancer patients was due to a greater proportion of premature births or whether the babies were small for gestational age, the distribution of birth weight percentiles (compensated for gestational age) was compared between the study and control groups. This analysis shows that babies born to women with breast cancer are significantly more likely to have a lower birth weight percentile ($p < 0.025$). Similarly, babies born to women with breast cancer were significantly more likely to be below the 50th percentile ($p < 0.009$) (Table 8.4).

The ratio of stillbirths to live births in our study (2 to 85, 2.4%) appears larger than in the general figure in Ontario (11.1 stillbirths in 1000 total births)[11]; however, this difference was not statistically significant. To further verify whether this tendency represents a true risk for stillbirth, we analyzed all 223 births occurring to women who had any form of cancer in PMH during the same 30 years. There were 10 stillbirths out of the 223 deliveries, a significantly greater ratio than in the population of Ontario ($p < 0.0005$). This still-birth rate represents a 4.23 relative risk (95% CI 2.0 to 7.8).

Table 8.4. *Distribution of birth weight percentile in the study and control groups*

	n	< 25th %ile	25–50th %ile	50th–75th %ile	75–90th %ile	> 90th %ile
Cases[a]	47	12	15	3	10	7
Matched controls*	73	8	15	18	14	18

[a] p < 0.025.

Discussion

Since the occurrence of breast cancer during pregnancy is relatively rare (3% of all breast cancers), it is highly unlikely that prospective trials will ever be large enough to assess the effect of breast cancer and its treatment on maternal and fetal outcome. To date, most available studies have analyzed the effect of pregnancy by comparing the course of breast cancer in pregnant women to a cohort of unmatched controls, thus carrying a risk of bias due to unbalanced prognostic factors[7,12,13]. The few studies that employed a case control analysis were composed of a small number of patients[6,14–16]. We found no statistically significant difference in cause-specific survival between pregnant and nonpregnant women matched by age, stage, and year of diagnosis. However, our data reveal that a pregnant woman has 2.5-fold higher risk of being diagnosed with metastatic breast cancer and a decreased chance of diagnosis of stage 1. Because the prognosis of metastatic breast cancer is poor (Fig. 8.5), this observation means that pregnancy *per se* poses a risk to women suffering from breast cancer. Similar findings have been suggested by Clark and Reid[4], Nugent and O'Connell[7], and Ribeiro *et al*[13]. However, none of these studies employed matched controls to substantiate their hypotheses.

Torres and Mickal[17], and Donegan[18], have suggested that, during pregnancy, the tumor is stimulated by the elevated estrogen levels, implying that the tumors are estrogen receptor (ER)-positive. However, it has been shown that young women, pregnant or not, usually have ER-negative breast cancer[7]. ER-negative tumors have a biologically aggressive course and carry a poor prognosis[19]. Thus, theoretically it is conceivable that pregnancy, with its hormonal stimulation, should not affect the course of the disease. This suggestion is supported by the observation that after matching for tumor stage, our pregnant patients had identical survival to the nonpregnant controls. Furthermore, termination of pregnancy was not associated with improved survival.

                                             D. Zemlickis et al.

Our data suggest that pregnant women are at a higher risk of presenting with advanced disease because pregnancy impedes early detection. During pregnancy, a woman's body undergoes substantial physiological changes, including enlargement of the breasts, that make it more difficult to notice small lumps that forewarn of cancer[20]. It is probable that many women and possibly their physicians relate findings consistent with breast cancer to pregnancy-induced enorgement. It has been reported that the average delay from first symptoms to treatment exceeds five months[6].

A pregnant woman may wish to delay her treatment for fear of the effects on the unborn baby. Among the regimes used in the treatment of breast cancer, chemotherapy has by far the highest likelihood of adversely affecting the baby during embryogenesis[21,22]. The effects of general anesthesia and surgery on the fetus have been investigated by several researchers, and unless complications occur (e.g., shock, hyperthermia), they do not appear to increase fetal risk[23,24]. Radiotherapy has the potential of causing irreversible harm to the fetus when fetal dose is above 10 rad; however, when radiation is directed to the breast, fetal dose is lower than the teratogenic range by several orders of magnitude[25]. In our study we found no malformations either in women who delayed treatment or in those who did not delay treatment. However, our cohort did not have babies that were delivered who were exposed to chemotherapy during embryogenesis, when major malformations would occur. Babies exposed to cancer chemotherapy later in pregnancy do not appear to have a higher risk for dysmorphology[22,26].

Children born to women with breast cancer were significantly more likely to be preterm, mainly due to more often elective cesarian sections to allow earlier start of cancer therapy. Of importance, our data are the first to document small birth weight for gestational age associated with breast cancer, which may be explained by the disease itself, as well as by its treatment. The higher rate of stillbirth in pregnancy further suggests suboptimal intrauterine conditions; the association between small birthweight and stillbirth has long been recognized[27].

Because the risk of metastatic disease is higher during pregnancy, it is important that pregnant women are instructed to perform regular breast self-examinations or that physicians caring for them perform the examinations during prenatal visits, with particular attention to any changes not consistent with pregnancy. Although breast cancer screening and treatment has advanced in the 30 years covered by this study, we cannot dismiss the importance of our results.

Because of the higher risk for stillbirth and small birth weight, women with breast cancer should be followed closely by a high-risk obstetrical unit, to define the optimal time of delivery.

References

1. Haagenson CD, Stout AP: Carcinoma of the breast; criteria of operability. *Ann Surg* 1943; 118: 859–870.
2. Applewhite RP, Smith LR, DiVincenti R: Carcinoma of the breast associated with pregnancy and lactation. *Am Surg* 1973; 39: 101–4.
3. Haagenson CD: Cancer of the breast in pregnancy and during lactation. *Am J Obstet Gynecol* 1967; 98: 141–9.
4. Clark RM, Reid J: Carcinoma of the breast in pregnancy and lactation. *Int J Radiation* 1978; 4: 693–8.
5. Ribeiro GG, Palmer MK: Breast carcinoma associated with pregnancy: a clinician's dilemma. *Br Med J* 1977; 2: 1524–7.
6. Max MH, Klamer TW: Pregnancy and breast cancer. *South Med J* 1983; 76: 1088–90.
7. Nugent P, O'Connel TX: Breast cancer and pregnancy. *Arch Surg* 1985; 120: 1221–4.
8. Anderson JM. Mammary cancers and pregnancy. *Br Med J* 1979; 1: 1124–7.
9. Parente JT, Amsel M, Lerner R, Chinea F. Breast cancer associated with pregnancy. *Obstet Gynocol* 1988; 71(6): 861–4.
10. Hermanek P, Sobin LH (eds.) TNM classification of malignant tumours, 4th edn. Springer-Verlag, 1987: 93–9, New York.
10a. Brenner WE, Edelman DA, Hendricks CH: A standard of fetal growth for the United States of America. *Am J Obstet Gynecol* 1986; 126: 555–64.
11. Registrar General of Ontario: Province of Ontario Vital Statistics: Table E, "Summary of live births, live births to unmarried mothers and stillbirths, and rates, Ontario." vols 1960 to 1985.
12. King RM, Welch JS, Martin JK, Coulam CB: Carcinoma of the breast associated with pregnancy. *Surg Gynecol Obstet* 1985; 160: 228–32.
13. Ribeiro G, Jones DA, Jones M: Carcinoma of the breast associated with pregnancy. *Br J Surg* 1986; 73: 607–9.
14. Sahni K, Sanyal B, Agrawal MS, Pant GC, Khanna NN, Khanna S: Carcinoma of breast associated with pregnancy and lactation. *J Surg Oncol* 1981; 16: 167–73.
15. Aghadiuno PU, Ibeziako PA: Clinicopathologic study of breast carcinoma occurring during pregnancy and lactation. *Int J Gynecol Obstet* 1983; 21: 17–26.
16. Tretli S, Kvalheim G, Thoresen S, Host H: Survival of breast cancer patients diagnosed during pregnancy or lactation. *Br J Cancer* 1988; 58: 382–4.
17. Torres JE, Mickal A: Carcinoma of the breast in pregnancy. *Clin Obstet Gynecol* 1975; 18: 219–25.
18. Donegan WL: Breast cancer and pregnancy. *Obstet Gynecol* 1977; 50: 244–52.
19. Zinns JS: The association of pregnancy and breast cancer. *J Reprod Med* 1979; 22: 197–301.
20. Hornstein E, Skornick Y, Rozin R: The management of breast carcinoma in pregnancy and lactation. *J Surg Oncol* 1982; 21: 179–2.

21. Nicholson HO: Cytotoxic drugs in pregnancy: review of reported cases. *J Obstet Gynecol* 1968; 75: 307.
22. Sutcliffe SB: Treatment of neoplastic disease during pregnancy: maternal and fetal effects. *Clin Invest Med* 1985; 8: 333–8.
23. Schardein JL: Cancer chemotherapeutic agents. In *Chemically Induced Birth Defects*. (Schardein JL, ed.), 1985: 467, Marcel Dekker Inc., New York.
24. Doll DC, Rigenberg QS, Yarbo JW: Management of cancer during pregnancy. *Arch Intern Med* 1988; 14: 2058–64.
25. National council on radiation protection and measurements: *Medical Radiation Exposure of Pregnant and Potentially Pregnant Women*. NCRP Report No. 54: 32, 1979.
26. Nicholson HO: Cytotoxic drugs in pregnancy: review of reported cases. *J Obstet Gynecol Br Commonw* 1968; 75: 307–12.
27. Brenner WE, Edelman DA, Hendricks CH: A standard of fetal growth for the United States of America. *Am J Obstet Gynecol* 1976; 126: 555–64.

9

Maternal and fetal outcome following Hodgkin's disease in pregnancy

M. LISHNER, D. ZEMLICKIS, P. DEGENDORFER,
T. PANZARELLA, S. B. SUTCLIFFE AND
G. KOREN

Introduction

Because the peak incidence of Hodgkin's Disease (HD) is in the age range 20–40 years, its association with pregnancy is not uncommon, occurring in 1 : 1000-1 : 6000 deliveries[1]. Early studies reported a higher frequency of relapse and lower survival rates in HD patients who were pregnant[2]. Later publications rejected this conclusion, claiming that pregnancy neither exacerbates the disease nor adversely affects survival[3–8]. The view that pregnancy does not affect the course of Hodgkin's disease and the disease does not affect the course of pregnancy has become widely accepted and repeatedly stressed in reviews and textbooks[1,9,10]. However, this conclusion is based on single cases or a surprisingly small number of uncontrolled studies[5–8].

It is unlikely that prospective controlled studies will ever be undertaken to explore further the interaction between HD and pregnancy; therefore, we performed a historical cohort study to evaluate the influence of pregnancy on HD and that of HD on pregnancy among women treated at the Princess Margaret Hospital (PMH) between 1958 and 1984. To the best of our knowledge, this is the only controlled study of HD and pregnancy. In addition, this study is unique in providing information on fetal outcome.

Methods

All patients with histologically confirmed Hodgkin's disease, registered in the Princess Margaret Hospital between 1958 and 1984, were identified.

To study the effects of pregnancy on the course of HD, we matched women having HD in pregnancy to nonpregnant women with the disease. For each pregnant case, an attempt was made to identify three matched controls in the PMH data base according to the following criteria:

1. The control women had to be within two years of age of the pregnant cases at diagnosis and could not have been pregnant within 15 months prior to or 9 months after first treatment.
2. Controls had the same Ann Arbor stage of HD as cases at diagnosis[11].
3. Controls had the same presence or absence of B symptoms as cases at diagnosis (fever, night sweats, and/or weight loss of more than 10% of the original weight six months prior to first attendance).
4. Controls were diagnosed within two calendaric years of the associated case. It was assumed that controls would have similar staging procedures and treatment protocols as the cases if controls were of same age, stage, and calendaric year of diagnosis as the cases. The validity of this assumption was verified in a random sample of ten pregnant women and 23 controls and was true 96% of the time.

Data describing patient characteristics with HD including date of diagnosis, staging, and presence or absence of B symptoms were extracted from the charts of both cases and controls. Dates and types of treatment, including treatment delays, were also recorded. Obstetrical information, including date of conception, gestational age at diagnosis and at first treatment, complications in pregnancy and its outcome were also recorded.

For cases whose pregnancies continued to term or resulted in stillbirth, birth records were requested from the delivering hospital. For live births, sex and birth weight of the infant were recorded, as well as gestational age at delivery, type of delivery, fetal complications and congenital anomalies. For intrauterine death, date of diagnosis of the stillbirth and autopsy results were collected.

Results

Forty-eight women with HD and pregnancy were identified in the PMH data base between 1958 and 1984. Two women had two pregnancies, each fitting in the time frame of the study, resulting in 50 pregnancies in 48 women. The mean age of women with HD was 26.1 ± 4.9 years (median 25 years and a range of 18 to 38 years). Of the 50 pregnancies, 12 (24%) were diagnosed with HD before conception, 10 (20%) during pregnancy, and 27 (54%) were diagnosed after delivery or pregnancy termination. For one pregnancy, this information was unavailable.

Treatment modalities of the 48 women included radiotherapy alone ($n = 31$), chemotherapy alone ($n = 6$), and combined radiotherapy and chemotherapy ($n = 11$). Of those women diagnosed before or during the pregnancy ($n = 22$), 16 women received radiation while pregnant, 1

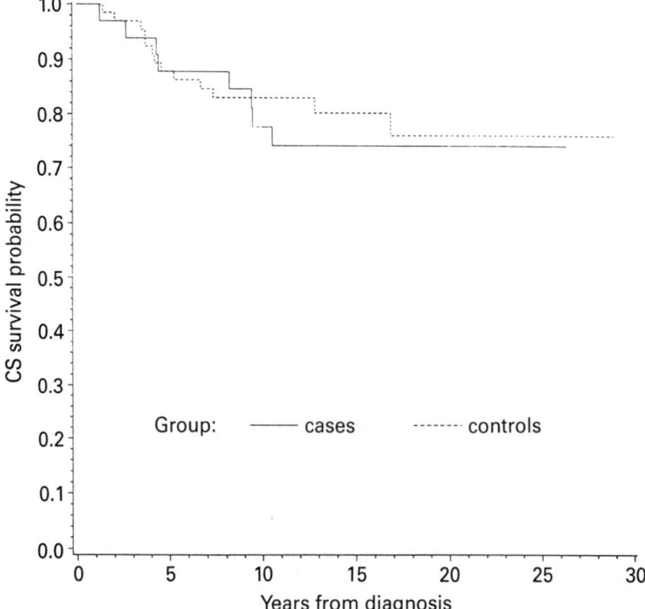

Fig. 9.1 Kaplan–Meier cause-specific survival curve for Hodgkin's Disease comparing women who were pregnant and had Hodgkin's Disease ($n = 33$) with matched, nonpregnant controls ($n = 67$). p = 0.6.

received chemotherapy during the first trimester, and 5 received combination chemotherapy and radiotherapy while pregnant. One patient delayed treatment due to pregnancy. She had received radiotherapy while pregnant and delayed chemotherapy until after delivery.

Of the 48 cases, 67 matched controls were found for 33 women. Three controls per patient could not always be obtained because of the selectivity of the matching criteria: for 15 cases, matched controls could not be found. This unmatched group was not statistically significantly different from the matched group when compared by survival (p = 0.6).

Maternal outcome

Using a cause-specific Kaplan–Meier survival curve, the 20-year survival of the 33 cases was compared to their 67 matched controls (Fig. 9.1). No statistically significant difference was found between these groups (p = 0.6). At the time of the study, 8 of the cases had died of HD while the remaining 25 were either alive or died of other causes. In the control group, 12 women died of HD.

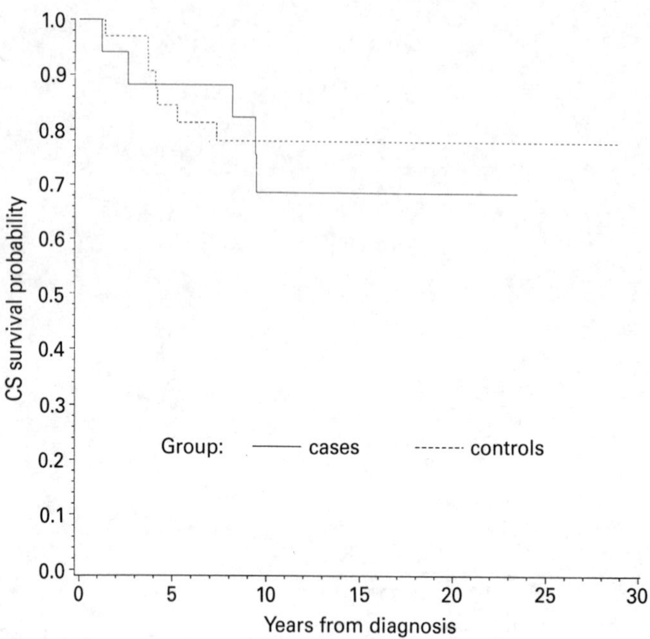

Fig. 9.2   Kaplan–Meier cause-specific survival curve for Hodgkin's disease comparing women who were diagnosed before or during pregnancy ($n = 17$) against their nonpregnant matched controls ($n = 33$). p = 0.6.

Fig. 9.2 compares survival in the subgroup of patients who were diagnosed with HD prior to conception or during the pregnancy and had matched controls ($n = 17$) with their nonpregnant matched controls ($n = 33$). No statistically significant difference in survival was found (p = 0.6). When the effect of individual stage of HD on maternal survival was analyzed, no significant differences were found between cases and controls (p > 0.1 for each comparison). To evaluate whether increasing age at diagnosis had an adverse impact on maternal cause-specific survival, we compared cases above ($n = 26$) to cases below ($n = 22$) the median age of 25 (Fig. 9.3). No statistically significant difference was found (p = 0.32).

In an attempt to verify whether pregnancy affected the stage of HD upon diagnosis, we compared the distribution of stages between our cases with that of nonpregnant women younger than 38 years registered in the PMH data base during the same time period (1958–1984). Of the 48 pregnant women, 12 (25%) had stage 1 disease at diagnosis, 22 (45.8%) stage 2, 8 (16.7%) stage 3, and 6 (12.5%) had stage 4. Of the 529 nonpregnant women identified in the computerized data base, 79 (15%) had stage 1 disease, 257

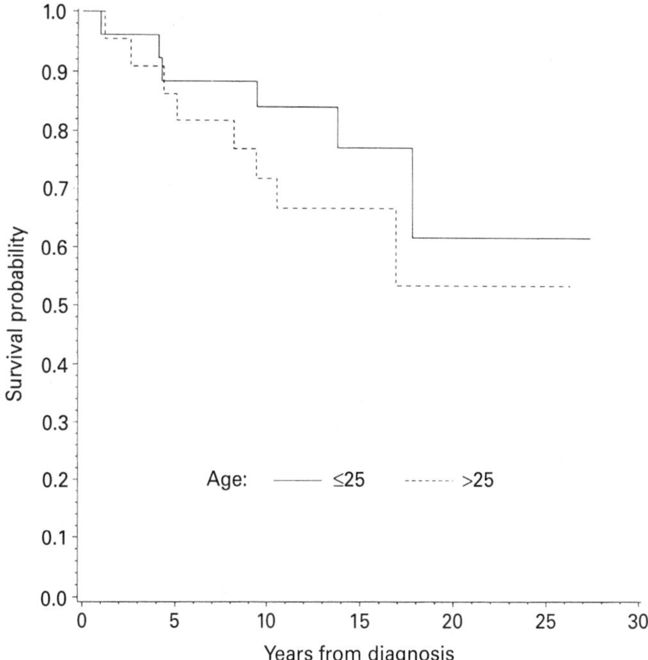

Fig. 9.3 Kaplan–Meier cause-specific survival curve for Hodgkin's Disease comparing women equal to or below the median age ($n = 26$) versus women above the median age ($n = 22$) of 25 years. p = 0.32.

(49%) stage 2, 106 (20%) stage 3, and 87 (16%) had stage 4. No statistically significant difference was found between these two distributions ($p > 0.25$).

Pregnancy outcome

Of the 50 pregnancies studied, there were 40 deliveries (2 of which were stillbirths), 5 miscarriages, and 4 therapeutic abortions. The outcome of 1 pregnancy was unknown.

Of the 38 live births, we were able to obtain 22 obstetrical records and 2 autopsy reports from the delivering hospitals (the remaining were unavailable due to unidentified delivering hospitals, destroyed birth records, or refusal to release confidential documents). However, in some additional cases, the maternal charts reported details of pregnancy outcome (Table 9.1).

No differences were found between the babies born to women with HD when compared to the Motherisk matched controls in birth weight ($p = 0.7$), mean gestational age ($p = 0.3$) or method of delivery ($p = 0.5$). One malformation was identified: this was a child with hydrocephaly born

Table 9.1. *Comparison of fetal outcome in mothers with Hodgkins disease to the matched control group (n = 38)*[a]

	Study babies		Matched control babies	
	n		n	
Gestational age (weeks)	29	39.7 ± 1.0	37	40.0 ± 1.8
Number of preterm births (< 37 weeks)	29	1	37	1
Birth weight (g)	21	3325 ± 529	37	3371 ± 474
Delivery method	25	20 spontaneous 5 cesarean	38	32 spontaneous 6 cesarean
Malformations	31	1 case of hydrocephaly, baby died 4 hours after birth	38	None
Stillbirth	40	2	38	None

[a] Plus-minus values are means $\pm$ SD.

to a mother whose HD was diagnosed before conception. She was treated only by combination chemotherapy (MOPP: nitrogen mustard, oncovin, prednisone, procarbazine) during the first trimester.

Of the 22 babies born and exposed to HD therapy *in utero*, one was exposed to chemotherapy during the first trimester of pregnancy, one was exposed to chemotherapy and radiation after the first trimester, 6 were exposed to radiation during the first trimester of pregnancy, and 17 were exposed to radiation after the first trimester.

We compared the number of stillbirths in our group (2 per 40 total births) to that of the general population of Ontario (11.3 stillbirths per 1000 total births) (Province of Ontario Vital Statistics, 1960–1984). The difference was not statistically significant ($p = 0.076$). To verify further whether this tendency represents a true risk for stillbirth, we analyzed all 223 births occurring to women who had any form of cancer in PMH during the same 30 years (Zemlickis *et al*). There were 10 stillbirths out of the 223 deliveries, a significantly greater ratio than in the population of Ontario ($p < 0.0005$). This stillbirth rate represents a 4.23 relative risk (95% CI 2.0 to 7.8).

Discussion

The diagnosis of HD in pregnancy puts immense stress on pregnant women, their families and on physicians caring for them. Potential harm to the woman from delayed diagnosis, staging or therapy, and the risk to the baby from radiation or chemotherapy creates immense pressure and a need for prompt decisions. For such choices to be authoritative, they must be based on large experience, which is lacking in any particular center owing to the relative rareness of the combination of HD and pregnancy.

Most published studies suffer from major problems that make them difficult to interpret and cast doubt on their validity. First, some of the frequently referenced studies were performed decades ago[3,5,12–14]. Since the diagnostic tools, staging methods, and especially treatment modalities have progressed tremendously in recent years, it is difficult to extrapolate these results to the present time. Secondly, most studies do not compare matched controls but rather compare pregnant women with a nonmatched cohort of nonpregnant women with HD[5,6]. Such reports carry a substantial risk of bias since the groups compared may be unbalanced by significant prognostic factors and thus the analysis may be misleading. Finally, some papers provide case reports or a summary of an experience with a small number of patients[15–17]. Although these reports are important, they cannot be used as guidelines for a rational clinical approach for these patients.

In contrast to previous work, our study is the first to use a case-control method to study the outcome of pregnant women with HD. It is based on a substantial number of patients that were carefully matched for the recognized and important prognostic factors of HD[1]. In addition, patients and controls were staged according to modern recommendations.

Our study did not detect an effect of pregnancy on survival of women with HD, as their long-term prognosis was identical to that of their matched controls. Moreover, this analysis reveals that the pregnant woman is not more likely to be at a higher stage (more advanced disease) than women of reproductive age in general. This indicates that pregnancy is not likely to change the biology of the tumor or to postpone diagnosis. These results are in contrast to our findings with breast cancer, where pregnant women have a significantly higher risk of being diagnosed with metastatic disease (stage 4)[18].

Our study is the first to provide data regarding fetal outcome by analyzing infants born to women with HD during pregnancy. We found that infants born to women with HD did not have a higher risk for prematurity or intrauterine growth retardation. Conversely, babies born to women with breast cancer have been shown by us to suffer from a significant small for gestational age (SGA) risk[18]. The rate of stillbirth was not statistically different from data for Ontario. This may reflect a beta error due to a small sample size, and larger numbers will be needed to confirm it.

                                                    M. Lishner et al.

Some authors recommend that patients who present in early pregnancy with HD should have a therapeutic abortion[9,16]. This recommendation is based on the potential harm of staging procedures, chemotherapy, or radiotherapy to the fetus[19,20]. However, we believe that recommendations regarding abortion should be individualized. Most patients in this study presented with an early stage disease. In these cases, HD can often be controlled and even cured with radiotherapy. Radiotherapy has the potential of causing irreversible harm to the fetus when fetal dose is above 10 rad[21]. However, when radiation is directed to the woman's neck (the most frequent presentation) fetal dose is lower than the teratogenic range by several orders of magnitude.

In contrast, when therapeutic doses must be delivered to the pelvis, therapeutic abortion seems justified. In patients who present with advanced disease, combined chemotherapy is the treatment of choice. Although various chemotherapeutic agents have been successfully administered during early pregnancy[8,22], there is compelling evidence that chemotherapy has significant likelihood of adversely affecting the baby during embryo genesis. The only infant in this series born to a patient who received chemotherapy during the first trimester (MOPP: nitrogen mustard, oncovin, prednisone, procarbazine) had hydrocephaly and died in early infancy. In contrast, there is no evidence for teratogenic effect of chemotherapy delivered during second or third trimester of pregnancy[19]. In our series, one baby was exposed to chemotherapy after the first trimester and was normal at birth. Much more data are needed to define the relative fetal risk of chemotherapy during embryogenesis as well as later.

In summary, this study could not detect adverse effects of pregnancy on survival of women with HD. Similarly, pregnant women are not likely to be at a higher stage of their disease than their matched controls. There is, however, a higher risk for stillbirth in women who have cancer, which should lead to follow-up of all such women by a high-risk perinatal unit. Decisions on the continuation of pregnancy and management of HD should be considered carefully and individually. This may ensure that most patients will be treated successfully without adversely affecting the outcome of either mother or infant.

References

1. Ward FT, Weiss RB: Lymphoma and pregnancy. *Sem Oncol* 1989; 16: 397–409.
2. Southman CM, Diamond HD, Craver LF: Hodgkin's disease in pregnancy.

Cancer 1956; 9(6): 1141–6.
3. Stewart HL, Monto RW: Hodgkin's disease and pregnancy. *Am J Obstet Gynecol* 1952; 63: 570–8.
4. Riva HL, Anderson PS, Grady GW: Pregnancy and Hodgkin's disease. A report of 8 cases. *Am J Obstet Gynecol* 1953; 66: 866–70.
5. Barry RM, Diamond HD, Craver LF: Influence of pregnancy on the course of Hodgkin's disease. *Am J Obstet Gynecol* 1962; 84: 445–54.
6. Gobbi PG, Attardo-Parrinello G, Danesimo M *et al*: Hodgkin's disease and pregnancy. *Hematologica* 1984; 69: 336–41.
7. Tawil E, Mercier JP, Dandarino A: Hodgkin's disease complicating pregnancy. *J Can Assoc Radio* 1985; 36: 133–7.
8. Nisce LZ, Tome MA, Shaogin H *et al*: Management of coexisting Hodgkin's disease and pregnancy. *Am J Clin Oncol* 1986; 9: 146–51.
9. Sutcliffe SB, Chapman RM: Lymphomas and leukemias. In: *Cancer in Pregnancy* (Allen HH, Nisker JA, ed.), 135. 1985, Futura Publishing Company Inc., Mt Kisco, New York.
10. Becker MH: Hodgkin's disease and pregnancy. *Radiol Clin N Am* 1968; VI: 111–14.
11. Hermanek P, Sobin LH: *TNM Classification of Malignant Tumours* 4th edn. 1987, pp. 175–179, Springer-Verlag, New York.
12. Kadson SC: Pregnancy and Hodgkin's disease: with a report of three cases. *Am J Obstet Gynecol* 1949; 57: 282–93.
13. Bichel J: Hodgkin's disease and pregnancy. *Acta Radiol* 1950; 33: 427–34.
14. Myles TJM: Hodgkin's disease and pregnancy. *J Obstet Gynecol Br Emp* 1955; 62: 844–91.
15. Howard LCDR, Smith N, Spaulding L: Hodgkin's disease and pregnancy. *South Med J* 1978; 71: 374–6.
16. Jacobs C, Donaldson SS, Rosenberg SI *et al*: Management of pregnant women with Hodgkin's disease. *Ann Intern Med* 1981; 95: 669–75.
17. Morgan OS, Hall JE, Gibbs WN: Hodgkin's disease in pregnancy. A report of three cases. *W I Med J* 1976; 25: 121–4.
18. Zemlickis D, Lishner M, Degendorfer P *et al*: Maternal and fetal outcome following breast cancer in pregnancy. *Am J Obstet Gynecol* 1992; 166: 781–7.
19. Koren G, Weiner L, Lishner M, Zemlickis D, Finegen J: Cancer in pregnancy: identification of unanswered questions on maternal and fetal risks. *Obstet Gynecol Surv* 1990; 45(8): 509–14.
20. Sweet DL, Kinzie J: Consequences of radiotherapy and antineoplastic therapy for the fetus. *J Reprod Med* 1976; 17: 241–6.
21. Becker MD, Hyman GA: Management of Hodgkin's disease coexistent with pregnancy. *Radiology* 1965; 85: 725–8.
22. Thomas PEM, Peckham JJ: The investigation and management of Hodgkin's disease in the pregnant patient. *Cancer* 1976; 38: 1443–51.

10

Non-Hodgkin's lymphoma and pregnancy

M. LISHNER, D. ZEMLICKIS, S. B. SUTCLIFFE
AND G. KOREN

Non-Hodgkin's lymphoma (NHL) has an age-dependent incidence pattern with a sharp increase in frequency starting in middle life[1]. In contrast, Hodgkin's disease (HD) exhibits a bimodal peak distribution. The first, in early adulthood, is followed by a plateau and a second peak after age 55[2]. These differences in age distributions together with the higher incidence of NHL in young males[1] probably explain the sparsity of reports of NHL associated with pregnancy in comparison with HD. These reports comprise mostly single cases[3,4] or a very small number of uncontrolled studies[5]. Thus, experience in the management of pregnancy complicated by NHL is limited and whether each of them affects the course of the other is still debated.

A careful review of published cases suggests that aggressive histology NHL is the most common type reported in pregnant patients[5-7]. This histologic presentation, the possible teratogenicity of some diagnostic methods and the possible benefit of some combined chemotherapy regimens (see below) dictate a limited staging workup during pregnancy. In addition, it is well established that tomographic scans and isotope studies are contraindicated during pregnancy due to potential harm to the fetus[5-9]. However, in contrast, abdominal ultrasound is safe and useful in pregnancy[10], while the role and safety of magnetic resonance imaging in the evaluation of pregnant women with NHL are still unclear[11]. Accordingly, it has been suggested that staging should include history, physical examination, routine blood tests bone marrow biopsies, chest X-ray with abdominal shielding and abdominal ultrasound[5].

Ward and Weiss summarized treatment results of 42 cases of NHL reported prior to 1990 in whom enough data were provided[5]. They report that 29 of these women died of lymphoma or complications of treatment while 11 were in remission at the time of the report and two were alive with signs of active disease. Analysis of the original studies shows that most surviving women either received combined aggressive chemotherapy or in rare cases had limited disease that could potentially be cured by local treatment which was either irradiation or surgery. It is possible that some women received treatment that enabled prolongation of life until after delivery of the fetus but was too conservative to achieve cure and indeed they documented 16 surviving infants in these 42 women. Thus, although the data available in the literature are limited, it seems that most patients should probably be treated with aggressive combination chemotherapy.

Aviles *et al*[7] recently described their experience with 16 pregnant women with NHL treated with combined chemotherapeutic regimens. They reported that 8 women achieved prolonged disease free survival and are currently considered cured. They also reported on 15 babies followed up for 3 to 11 years who are all alive and well, although eight of the mothers were treated in the first trimester of pregnancy. Nevertheless, it should be remembered that, despite the fact that various chemotherapeutic agents have been successfully administered during early pregnancy[9], there is still compelling evidence that cancer chemotherapy has a substantial potential of adversely affecting embryogenesis[12,13]. Chemotherapy during the first trimester may expose the embryo to toxicity potentially capable of producing embryonic death or major malformations[14]. Approximately 10% of patients exposed to cytotoxic drugs during the first trimester of pregnancy exhibit major malformations[15]. In contrast, there is no evidence for the teratogenic effect of chemotherapy delivered during the second or third trimesters of pregnancy[13,15]. In addition, the rate of fetal malformation after a combination of cytotoxic drugs in the first trimester is only slightly higher than the rate observed with a single agent[16].

The rare pregnant women presenting with either low grade or localized, intermediate grade lymphoma should be treated by more conservative approaches based on individual decision making in each case. Two additional points should be stressed. First, the course of Burkitt's lymphoma and lymphoblastic lymphoma among pregnant women has been reported to be lethal[5,12]. However, the cases reported over the last decades are difficult to interpret because patients were treated using different approaches and chemotherapeutic agents and the survival could probably be enhanced with appropriate modern management[12]. Secondly Steiner-Salz *et al* observed rapid clinical progression of aggressive NHL during the immediate post partum period[17], while Sutcliffe and Chapman concluded from their experience that pregnancy does not seem to affect the course of lymphoma[18].

Our own series includes ten women with histologically proven NHL and pregnancy registered in the Princess Margaret Hospital database between 1958 and 1984. The mean age was 26.6 ($\pm$ 8.6) years. Two were diagnosed with NHL just before conception, three during pregnancy and five after delivery or termination of the pregnancy. Of the ten women, four received radiotherapy as their first treatment modality, two received chemotherapy and four received radiation and chemotherapy. The cause-specific survival at 10 years was 67%. Of the three women who were treated during pregnancy, one received radiation during the second trimester. The other two were treated with chemotherapy, one in the first and the other in the second trimester. The two latter patients have been reported previously. Of the ten pregnancies there were seven live births, one therapeutic abortion, one spontaneous abortion and in another case it is still unknown whether the mother had a spontaneous or therapeutic abortion. We were able to obtain five obstetrical reports from the delivering hospitals. Babies who were born to mothers who had NHL appeared to have a trend towards lower mean birthweight compared to their matched controls. However, this was not found to be statistically significant ($p = 0.09$) probably due to the small sample size.

In summary, the diagnosis of NHL in pregnancy puts immense stress on pregnant women, their families and on the physicians taking care of them. Potential harm to the women from delays in diagnosis, staging or therapy on the one hand, and the risk to the baby from radiation or chemotherapy on the other, creates serious pressure on all concerned and a need for prompt decisions. However, the decision-making process is complicated by the existence of only sparse data on both the maternal and fetal outcome. Based on small series and case reports, it seems that most lymphomas complicating pregnancy are of the aggressive type and disseminated in nature. Although the prognosis had been reported to be poor, there is evidence to suggest that pregnancy does not affect the course of lymphoma when properly treated. We believe that aggressive chemotherapy, when indicated, can be delivered during pregnancy after proper counseling of the pregnant woman and her family. Rare localized or low grade lymphomas should be treated individually with a more conservative approach. Large, controlled, multicenter studies are still needed in the future in order to evaluate the effect of pregnancy on the course of the NHL and that of the malignant disease and its treatment on the mother and her offspring.

References

1. Jandle JH: Non-Hodgkin's lymphoma. In *Blood: Textbook of Hematology*, (Jandle JH, ed.) 1987, pp. 891–964, Little, Brown and Company, Boston/Toronto.
2. Gutensohn NY, Cole P: Epidemiology of Hodgkin's disease. *Semin Oncol* 1980; 7: 92–102.
3. Ortega J: Multiple agent chemotherapy, including bleomycin, of non-Hodgkin's lymphoma during pregnancy. *Cancer* 1977; 40: 2829–35.
4. Spitzer M, Citron M, Ilardi QF, Saxe B: Case report: non-Hodgkin's lymphoma during pregnancy. *Gynecol Oncol* 1991; 43: 309–12.
5. Ward FT, Weiss RB: Lymphoma in pregnancy: three cases and review of the literature. *Arch Pathol Lab Med* 1989; 109: 803–9.
6. Joachim HL: Non-Hodgkin's lymphoma in pregnancy: three cases and review of the literature. *Arch Pathol Lab Med* 1985; 109: 803–9.
7. Aviles A, Diaz-Maguco JC, Torras V *et al*: Non-Hodgkin's lymphoma and pregnancy: presentation of 16 cases. *Gynecol Oncol* 1990; 37: 335–7.
8. Donegan WL: Cancer and pregnancy. *CA* 1983; 33: 194–214.
9. Nisce LZ, Tome MA, He S *et al*: Management of co-existing Hodgkin's disease and pregnancy. *Am J Clin Oncol* 1968; 9: 146–51.
10. Anderson TM, Lee TG, Nagel N: Ultrasound diagnosis of nonobstetric disease during pregnancy. *Obst Gynecol* 1976; 48: 359–62.
11. Consensus Conference: Magnetic resonance imaging. *J Am Med Assoc* 1988; 259: 2132–8.
12. Darnell Jones DE, d'Avignon MB, Lawrence R, Latshow RF: Burkitt's lymphoma: obstetric and gynecologic aspects. *Obstet Gynecol* 1980; 56: 533–63.
13. Lishner M, Koren G: *Fetal Risk of Cancer Chemotherapy in Pregnancy*. (Allen HH, Nisker JA, Sutcliffe SB, ed.), 1993, Futura Publishing Company Inc. Mt. Kisco, New York (in press).
14. Sutcliffe SB: Treatment of neoplastic disease during pregnancy: maternal and fetal effects. *Clin Invest Med* 1985; 8: 333–8.
15. Koren G, Weiner L, Lishner, M. *et al*: Cancer and pregnancy: identification of unanswered questions on maternal and fetal risks. *Obstet Gynecol Surv* 1990; 45: 509–14.
16. Doll DC, Ringenberg QS, Yarbo JW: Management of cancer during pregnancy. *Arch Int Med* 1988; 14: 2058–64.
17. Steiner-Salz D, Yahalom J, Samuelov A, Polliack A: Non-Hodgkin's lymphoma associated with pregnancy. A report of six cases with a review of the literature. *Cancer* 1985; 56: 2087–91.
18. Sutcliffe SB, Chapman RM: Lymphomas and leukemias. In *Cancer in Pregnancy* (Allen HH, Nisker JA, ed.), 1986, pp. 135–189. Futura, Mt. Kisco.

11

Maternal and fetal outcome following invasive cervical cancer in pregnancy

M. LISHNER, D. ZEMLICKIS, P. DEGENDORFER,
T. PANZARELLA, S. B. SUTCLIFFE AND
G. KOREN

Introduction

Invasive carcinoma of the cervix is the most common gynecological malignancy associated with pregnancy because of its tendency to occur in the reproductive years[1]. However, its occurrence is rare with an incidence of approximately 1 per 1240–2200 pregnancies[2,3]. Although the relationship between carcinoma of the cervix and pregnancy has been extensively studied, review of the literature reveals that most studies were based on case reports[4], cohorts whose controls were not matched on prognostic factors[3], and cohorts without a control group[5–7].

Since it is unlikely that prospective studies will be conducted, due to the rarity of cervical cancer in pregnancy, we performed a matched historical cohort study to evaluate the influence of pregnancy on cervical cancer and cervical cancer on pregnancy, among women treated in the Princess Margaret Hospital in Toronto between 1958 and 1984. In addition, information regarding fetal outcome is provided.

Methods

All women with histologically confirmed invasive carcinoma of the cervix registered in the Princess Margaret Hospital from 1958 (when the hospital opened) to 1984 (when pregnancy was no longer in the data base) were identified.

To evaluate the effects of pregnancy on the course of the cervical cancer we matched women with the disease in pregnancy to nonpregnant women with carcinoma of the cervix. For each case, an attempt was made to identify three matched controls in the PMH's data base according to the following criteria:

120

1. The control women had to be within two calendaric years of age of the cases at diagnosis and could not have been pregnant at any time from 15 months prior to first treatment to 9 months after first treatment.
2. Controls were diagnosed within two calendaric years of the associated case.
3. Controls had the same clinical TNM and clinical stage (FIGO) of carcinoma of cervix as cases at diagnosis[8,9].

The date of diagnosis and stage of cancer were extracted from the charts of both cases and controls. Stages were grouped according to the TNM classification[9]. Dates and types of treatment including treatment delays were also recorded. Obstetrical information including date of conception, gestational age at diagnosis and first treatment, complications of pregnancy if any, mode of delivery and fetal outcome were also extracted.

For cases whose pregnancies continued to term or resulted in stillbirths, birth records were requested from the delivering hospital. For live births, sex and birth weight of the infants were recorded as well as gestational age at delivery, type of delivery, fetal complications and congenital anomalies. For intrauterine death, date of diagnosis of the stillbirths and autopsy results were requested.

Results

Forty women with invasive carcinoma of the cervix with an associated pregnancy were registered in the PMH's data base between 1958 and 1984. The average age at diagnosis was 34.0 ± 5.9 years (median age 34, range 21 to 45). Of the 40 pregnancies, 23 women were diagnosed with cervical cancer during pregnancy and the remaining 17 were diagnosed after delivery or termination of the pregnancy.

Of the 40 women, 14 had surgery as first treatment, 23 received external radiation with or without intracavitary radium insertion, 1 had only intracavitary radium insertion, 1 had surgery and external radiation, and 1 received all three treatments. Of the 23 women diagnosed during pregnancy, there were 12 therapeutic abortions, 2 miscarriages, 9 live births (1 pregnancy resulted in twins), and 1 stillbirth. Six women chose to delay the recommended treatment until after delivery of a live birth (in four cases) or stillbirth (one case), or termination (one case) of the pregnancy. Of the four deliveries where treatment was not delayed, the babies were born by immediate cesarean section because diagnosis was made in the third trimester, followed by treatment. Only three babies were exposed *in utero* to external radiation; all three women chose to therapeutically terminate the pregnancy.

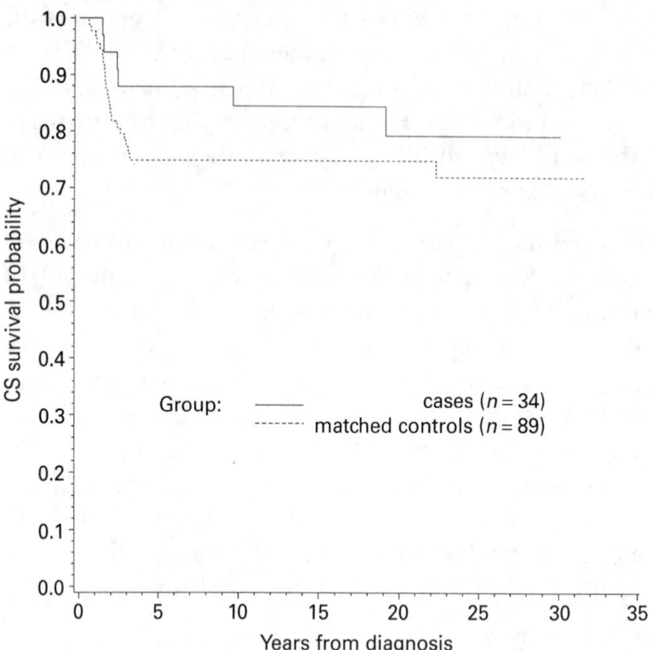

Fig. 11.1   Kaplan–Meier cause-specific survival curve comparing women who were pregnant and had invasive cervical cancer ($n = 34$) against matched nonpregnant controls ($n = 89$). p = 0.31.

There were 89 matched controls identified for 34 cases. Three controls per patient could not always be obtained because the matching criteria were selective enough that the PMH patient data base did not always contain three matches per case. To ensure that the groups were indeed similar, we compared the distribution of the matching criteria within them. As expected, no significant difference was found ($p > 0.25$ for each test). Six cases did not have matched controls; five patients were diagnosed with cervical cancer during the early 1960s and could not be matched because computer records at that time contained ambiguous staging codes. The remaining patient could not be matched because she could not be properly staged. Review of these six charts did not reveal any systematic features that would explain why these patients could not be matched.

Using a Kaplan–Meier cause-specific survival curve, the 30-year survival of the 34 cases was compared to their 89 matched controls (Fig. 11.1). No statistically significant difference was found between the two groups ($p = 0.31$). At the time of the study, 6 of the cases had died of cervical cancer while the remaining 28 were either alive or died of other causes. In the control group, 22 women died of cervical cancer.

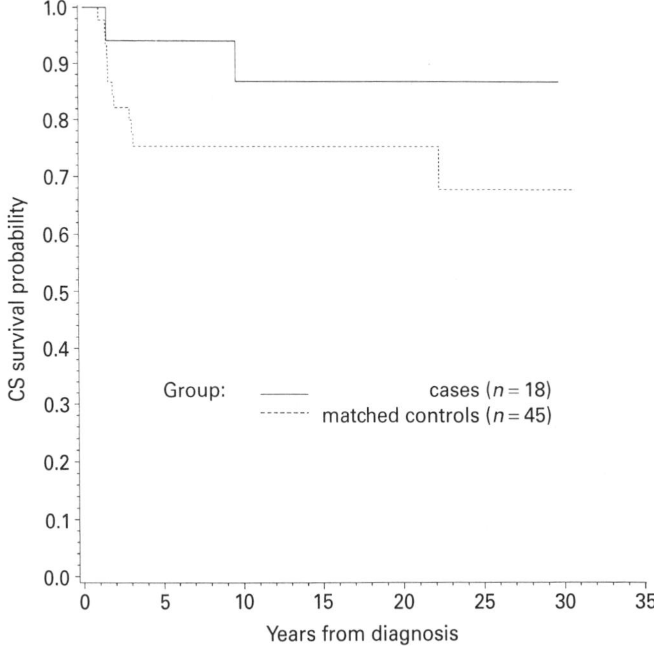

Fig. 11.2 Kaplan–Meier cause-specific survival curve. The survival of women who were diagnosed with invasive cervical cancer before or during their pregnancy ($n = 18$) is compared to their nonpregnant matched controls ($n = 45$). p = 0.22.

Fig. 11.2 compares the survival of the subgroup of 18 patients diagnosed with cancer during pregnancy with their 45 matched controls. No statistically significant difference was found (p = 0.22).

The distribution by clinical stage and trimester of pregnancy at the time of diagnosis is presented in Table 11.1. For women who were diagnosed with cervical cancer during pregnancy, eight were diagnosed during the first trimester, nine during the second, and six during the third. No statistically significant difference was found in maternal survival between the three trimesters (p = 0.68, Fig. 11.3).

In an attempt to verify whether pregnancy affected the stage of cervical cancer upon diagnosis, we compared the distribution of stages in our cases with that of nonpregnant women younger than 45 years registered in the PMH data base diagnosed during the same time period (1958–1984). Of the 39 pregnant women with available staging, 27 (69%) had stage 1 disease at diagnosis, 9 (23%) stage 2, and 3 (8%) had stage 3. Of the 1963 women identified in the computerized data base, 825 (42%) were diagnosed with stage 1 disease, 681 (35%) with stage 2, 410 (21%) with stage 3, and 47 (2%)

Table 11.1. *Distribution of clinical stage with trimester of pregnancy on diagnosis of cancer (n = 40)*

Trimester	Stage 1 ($n = 27$)	Stage II ($n = 9$)	Stage III ($n = 3$)	Unknown ($n = 1$)
1 ($n = 8$)	5	1	1	1
2 ($n = 9$)	6	2	1	0
3 ($n = 6$)	5	1	0	0
Postpartum ($n = 17$)	11	5	1	0

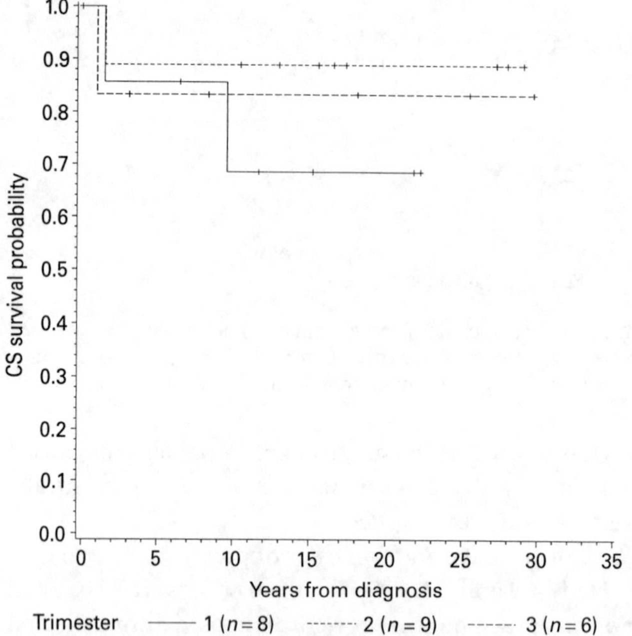

Fig. 11.3   Kaplan–Meier cause-specific survival curve. Survival is compared for women who were diagnosed with invasive cervical cancer during the first ($n = 8$), second ($n = 9$), and third ($n = 6$) trimesters. p = 0.68.

with stage 4. This distribution is statistically significantly different from that of the pregnant women (p < 0.005). When analyzed by individual stage, and adjusted for multiple comparisons (Bonferroni method), a statistically higher number of women were diagnosed with stage 1 disease in the pregnant group as compared to the PMH data base (p = 0.0006). The relative risk of having stage 1 disease in pregnancy is 3.1 (95% CI of 1.6 to 6.2). The number of women who had stages 3 and 4 in the pregnant group (3, 7.7%) appears smaller than the number in the PMH data base (457,

Table 11.2. *Types of treatment by clinical stage of disease (n = 40)*

Stage	Surgery	External radiation[a]	Other
I	12	13	2
II	2**	7	0
III	0	2	1
Unknown	0	1	0

[a]External radiation with or without intracavitary radium.
[b]Two patients received surgery for stage 2 cervical cancer when radiation is the treatment of choice. These women were diagnosed and treated in 1959 and 1967.

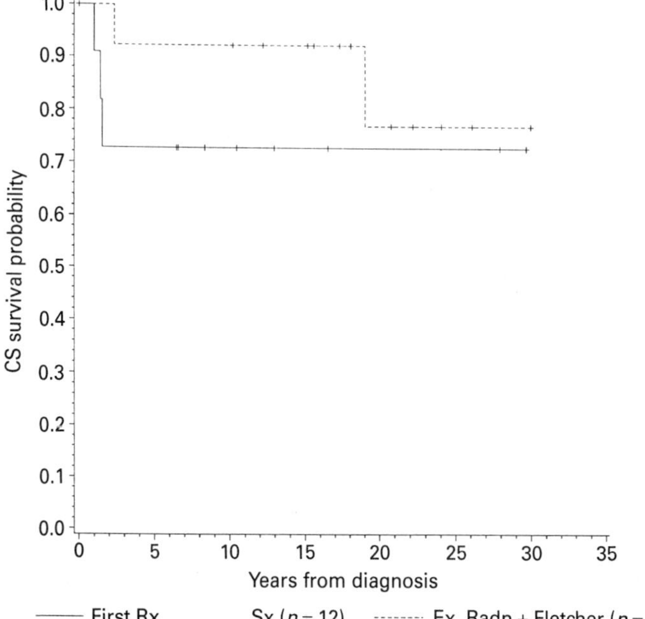

Fig. 11.4   Kaplan–Meier cause-specific survival curve. Survival of women with stage 1 invasive cervical cancer was compared between women who had surgery ($n = 12$) and women who had external radiation with or without intracavitary radium insertion ($n = 13$). p = 0.3.

23.3%). This distribution was statistically significant after adjusting for multiple comparisons (p = 0.02).

The distribution of treatment modalities in the study women by stage at diagnosis is provided in Table 11.2. Cause-specific survival was used to compare patients with stage 1 disease by mode of treatment (Fig. 11.4). No statistically significant difference was found between the 12 women who

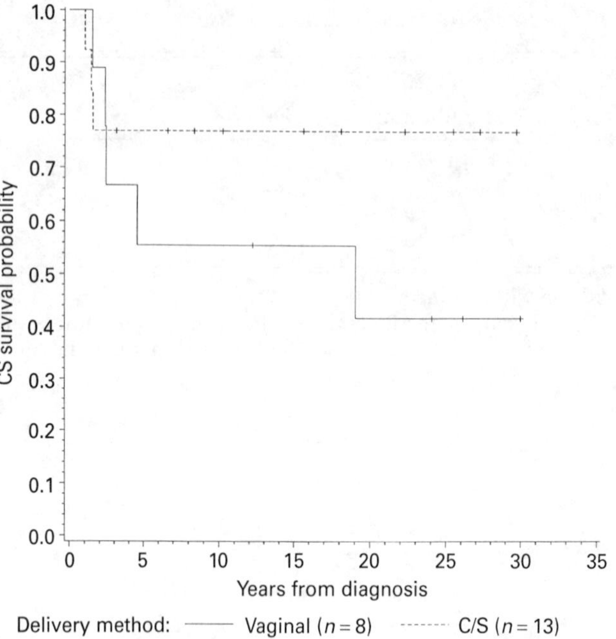

Fig. 11.5 Kaplan–Meier cause-specific survival curve comparing women with invasive cervical cancer who delivered spontaneously ($n = 8$) to those women who had a cesarean section ($n = 13$). p = 0.3.

had surgery and the 13 women who had external radiation with or without intracavitary radium insertion (p = 0.3).

In an attempt to verify whether vaginal delivery hastens dissemination of invasive cervical cancer, we compared maternal survival by delivery method for the 21 women for whom delivery information was available. The cause-specific survival curve (Fig. 11.5) showed no statistically significant difference between the 8 women who delivered spontaneously and the 13 who had cesarean section (p = 0.3), although there was a trend for better survival with the latter.

Fetal outcome

Of the 40 pregnancies studied, there were 12 therapeutic abortions, 4 miscarriages, and 24 deliveries. Of the 24 deliveries, there were 23 live births and 2 stillbirths.

Of the 24 deliveries, we received 13 obstetrical records and 1 autopsy report from the delivery hospital. The remaining records could not be

Table 11.3. *Comparison of fetal outcome in mothers with invasive cervical cancer to the matched control group (n = 21)*[a]

	Study babies		Matched control babies	
	n		*n*	
Gestational age (weeks)	19	37.2 ± 44[c]	21	39.2 ± 2.1[c]
Preterm births (< 37 weeks)	19	3	21	2
Birth weight (g)	12	2799 ± 768[b]	21	3338 ± 644[b]
Delivery method	21	8 spontaneous 13 cesarean	21	16 spontaneous 5 cesarean
Malformations	23	None	21	None
Stillbirths	25	2	21	None

[a]Plus–minus values are means ± SD.
[b]p = 0.04.
[c]p = 0.09.

obtained because delivering hospitals were unknown or birth records were destroyed or unavailable to us due to confidentiality policies of the delivering hospitals. However, some maternal charts did report details of the pregnancy. A summary of the available information regarding fetal outcome is presented in Table 11.3.

There was no statistically significant difference in mean gestational age (p = 0.09) or in the proportion of preterm births (p = 0.7). There was a statistically lower mean birth weight for babies of mothers with invasive cervical cancer when compared to their matched controls (p = 0.04).

To assess whether the lower birth weight in babies of cancer patients was due to a greater proportion of cesarean sections or due to intrauterine growth restriction (IUGR), the distribution of birth weight percentiles (compensated for gestational age) was compared between the study and control groups. By comparing the proportion of babies born above and below the 50th percentile[10], we show that babies born to women with invasive cervical cancer are not significantly more likely to have a lower birth weight percentile (p = 0.3) (Table 11.4).

The ratio of stillbirths to live births in the study group (2 per 25 total births) was compared to that of the general population of Ontario (11.1 stillbirths per 1000 total births)[11]. This difference did not reach statistical significance. To verify whether this tendency represents a true risk for stillbirth, we analyzed all 223 births occurring to women who had any form of cancer in PMH during the same 30 years[12]. There were 10 stillbirths out

Table 11.4. *Distribution of birth weight percentile in the study and control groups*

	n	Birth weight percentile for gestational age at delivery (%)					
		< 10	10–25	25–50	50–75	75–90	> 90
Cases[a]	12	2	1	4	3	1	1
Matched controls[a]	21	3	0	5	3	5	5

[a] $p = 0.30$.

of the 223 deliveries, a significantly greater ratio than in the population of Ontario ($p < 0.0005$). This stillbirth rate represents a 4.23 relative risk (95% CI of 2.0 to 7.8).

Discussion

The diagnosis of invasive cervical cancer in pregnancy poses a difficult challenge to the woman, her family, and the physicians caring for her. Maternal survival may be compromised due to delayed diagnosis or treatment. The mother may find it necessary to therapeutically terminate the pregnancy to hasten treatment or may miscarry because of treatment. These decisions may be particularly difficult because the mother may face diminished reproductive function as a result of treatment. These decisions may be easier if based on the results of large prospective studies. However, as the incidence of invasive cervical cancer is rare (1 per 1240–2200 pregnancies), large prospective studies are impractical[2,3].

Most studies, to date, contain defects which make their results difficult to interpret reliably. Some studies were performed decades ago when diagnostic procedures and staging methods were significantly different making it difficult to relate their results to present-day cases[17,18]. Case reports or studies employing a very small sample size are difficult to interpret[4,7]. In some studies, the effect of pregnancy on cervical carcinoma was assessed by comparing the pregnant women with control groups that were not matched for maternal age or year of diagnosis[3,2]. Such an analysis carries a risk of bias since the groups analyzed may have unbalanced prognostic factors, or different surgical and radiation techniques may have been used. Some studies have not employed control groups, making it very difficult to determine the impact of pregnancy[5–7]. In contrast, we believe our study is the first to employ controls matched for established prognostic factors.

Our study indicates that there is no difference in maternal survival between women who are pregnant with cervical cancer with nonpregnant women matched by age, stage, and year of diagnosis. However, our results demonstrate that a pregnant woman has a 3.1-fold higher chance of being diagnosed with stage 1 cervical cancer. This demonstrates that pregnancy-related obstetrical examinations are effective and essential for early detection.

In a previous study by our group concerning breast cancer in pregnancy, we have shown that pregnant women have a 2.5-fold increased risk to present with metastatic breast cancer due to late diagnosis[12]. This result, combined with our present conclusion that early detection results in presentation of an early stage of cervical cancer, further highlights the importance of early diagnosis of cancer in the pregnant woman.

We found no difference in maternal survival between women who have a vaginal delivery or cesarean section, agreeing with the results of McNulty and Roberts[15] and Hacker *et al*[2].

For the purposes of this paper, intrauterine growth restriction (IUGR) is defined as a fetus whose weight is abnormally low for its gestational age. In contrast to our earlier findings of IUGR associated with breast cancer[12], we found no statistically significant difference in the distribution of birth weight percentiles between babies born to women with cervical cancer and the Motherisk control group. It is important to observe that the gestational age of our cohort was not statistically different from that of the Motherisk control group. However, we did observe a higher percentage of cesarean sections in the cancer group compared to the Motherisk group.

Surgery and radiation are the treatments of choice for nonmetastatic, nonrecurrent invasive cervical cancer. Both forms of treatment will cause termination of pregnancy. In our study, six women delayed treatment until after delivery or termination of the pregnancy. No delivered babies were exposed to any form of therapy *in utero*. It has been suggested that there exists a difference in maternal survival between treatment by surgery or radiation for stage 1 cervical cancer[2]. We, in agreement with other authors, have found no evidence to substantiate this claim[16].

In summary, this study provides evidence that pregnancy does not adversely affect survival of women with invasive cervical cancer. Because pregnant women are likely to have better gynecological follow-up than nonpregnant women with cervical cancer, early diagnosis assures less disseminated disease. Because of the risk of stillbirth, women with invasive cervical cancer should be followed closely by a high-risk obstetrical unit to define the optimal time of delivery.

References

1. Jolles CJ: Gynecologic cancer associated with pregnancy. *Sem Oncol* 1989; 16: 417–24.
2. Hacker NF, Berek JCC, Lagasse LD *et al*: Carcinoma of the cervix associated with pregnancy. *Obstet Gynecol* 1982; 59: 735–46.
3. Lee RB, Neglia W, Park RC: Cervical carcinoma in pregnancy. *Obstet Gynecol* 1981; 58: 584–9.
4. Saunders N, Landon CR: Management problems associated with carcinoma of the cervix diagnosed in the second trimester of pregnancy. *Gynecol Oncol* 1988; 30: 120–2.
5. LaVecchi C, Franceschi S, DeCarli A *et al*: Invasive cervical cancer in young women. *Br J Obstet Gynecol* 1984; 91: 1149–55.
6. Nisker JA, Shubat M: Stage 1B cervical carcinoma and pregnancy: report of 49 cases. *Am J Obstet Gynecol* 1983; 145(2): 203–6.
7. Funnell JD, Puckett TG, Strebel GF, Kelso JW: Carcinoma of the cervix complicating pregnancy. *South Med J* 1980; 73(10): 1308–10.
8. International Federation of Gynecology and Obstetrics: Changes in definitions of clinical staging for carcinoma of the cervix and ovary. *Am J Obstet Gynecol* 1987; 153: 263.
9. Hermanek P, Sobin LH, (eds): *TNM Classification of Malignant Tumors*, 4th edn., pp. 104–107, 1987, Springer-Verlag, New York.
10. Brenner WE, Edelman DA, Hendricks CH: A standard of fetal growth for the United States of America. *Am J Obstet Gynecol* 1976; 126: 555–64.
11. Registrar General of Ontario: Province of Ontario Vital Statistics: Table E, "Summary of live births, live births to unmarried mothers and stillbirths, and rates, Ontario." Vols 1960 to 1984.
12. Zemlickis D, Lishner M, Degendorfer P *et al*: Maternal and fetal outcome following breast cancer in pregnancy. *Am J Obstet Gynecol* 1992; 166: 781–7.
13. Prem KA, Makowski EL, McKelvey JL: Carcinoma of the cervix associated with pregnancy. *Am J Obstet Gynecol* 1966; 95: 99–108.
14. Lash AF: Management of carcinoma of the cervix in pregnancy. *Obstet Gynecol* 1961; 17: 41–8.
15. McNulty B, Roberts WS: Elective cesarean hysterectomy versus vaginal hysterectomy for the treatment of cervical intraepithelial neoplasia. *South Med J* 1987; 80(8): 984–6.
16. Lutz MH, Underwood PB, Rozier JC, Putney FW: Genital malignancy in pregnancy. *Am J Obstet Gynecol* 1977; 129: 536–42.

12
Pregnancy and ovarian cancer

M. LISHNER, D. ZEMLICKIS AND G. KOREN

Malignant ovarian neoplasms during pregnancy are exceedingly rare with an incidence of 1 : 10000–1 : 100000 term deliveries[1,2]. Most women are in their third decade of life at the time of tumor detection. It has been suggested that pregnancy and hormonal manipulations have a protective effect against ovarian cancer[3]. Furthermore, tumors detected during pregnancy are much less likely to be malignant when compared to those not occurring during gestation[4].

It has been observed that most ovarian neoplasms during pregnancy are detected on routine physical examination during first prenatal visit[2,5,6]. In contrast, other authors indicated that the majority of their patients were symptomatic at the time of presentation with abdominal pain, distention or acute intra-abdominal catastrophe such as torsion or rupture[7,8]. The high frequency of obstetric ultrasound scanning in current practice may increase the detection rate of ovarian tumors during pregnancy[2]. However, it has been shown that such tumors are not infrequently missed, especially in the second and third trimesters, since the growing uterus may conceal large tumors or ovarian neoplasms may not be separated from a cystic enlarged gravid uterus[1,2]. Although sonography is the primary imaging tool in pregnant women who present with pelvic mass, its specificity is low and many ovarian tumors that do not require intervention are detected. As computed tomography (CT), that uses ionizing radiation, is not desirable during pregnancy[9], magnetic resonance (MR) imaging can provide supplemental information that may influence patient treatment when results of sonography are equivocal[10].

Approximately two-thirds of ovarian cancers detected during pregnancy are of epithelial origin (as compared to 90% of ovarian tumors in the general population)[1,2]. In sharp contrast to the general population, most epithelial tumors during pregnancy are of low grade and low stage (usually stage 1)[4,7,9,10,11]. These two factors are powerful predictors of favorable outcome. Of the germ cell tumors which occur in younger women, dysgerminoma is the most common during pregnancy[9].

A detailed approach to management of ovarian cancer in pregnancy is beyond the scope of this chapter. It is generally believed that explorative laparotomy with frozen sections from any suspected lesion should be employed. The surgical approach can vary from a conservative to radical one depending on characteristics of the patient, the tumor and the gestation[2,12]. It is clear that conservative approach enables continuation of gestation and final decisions can be reached after delivery. Chemotherapy and/or radiotherapy are administered according to the findings in laparotomy. Since most ovarian cancers in pregnancy are epithelial and of low stage and grade, most women will not require termination of pregnancy[1]. Treatment of patients with higher stage or grade involves radical surgery complemented by radiotherapy and chemotherapy.

The effect of abdominal surgery on the course of pregnancy is controversial. A high risk of pregnancy loss associated with ovarian surgery in pregnancy, especially in the second trimester, has been reported[13,14]. Others claim that severe third trimester complications may result from failure to remove significant ovarian masses during mid-pregnancy and from performing surgery during the third trimester[15–17]. There seems to be a general agreement that operative intervention is indicated as soon as the diagnosis of ovarian tumor in pregnancy is made, irrespective of the age of pregnancy.

Our experience at the PMH includes 11 patients with ovarian cancer and pregnancy identified in the 30 years analyzed in our study. Their mean age was 27.5–7.1 (range 17–41) years. The 15-year survival rate is 64%. Of the 11 pregnancies there were nine live births, one therapeutic abortion and one stillbirth. The stillbirth, diagnosed at 24 weeks of gestation, was attributed to intrauterine anoxia secondary to mechanical compression of the umbilical cord by the ovarian mass. Four deliveries were complicated: one by severe respiratory distress syndrome, two by intrauterine infection and in one patient labor was probably precipitated by rupture of her ovarian tumor. The mean birth weight of babies born to mothers with ovarian cancers (2697 ± 766 g) was less than the mean birth weight of babies from the control group (3353 ± 476 g). However, the trend did not reach statistical significance. Additionally, there was no significant difference in the mean gestational age between the two groups (p = 0.11). Children born to mothers with ovarian cancer were often preterm, mainly because elective cesarean sections were performed to allow earlier start of cancer therapy.

In summary, it is conceivable that more ovarian masses in pregnancy are being detected lately. These masses should be managed just as in the nonpregnant patients. Pregnancy does not seem to affect the course of ovarian cancer. Since most ovarian cancers are of low grade and stage, prognosis is quite favorable, with five-year survival rate of 60–75%.

References

1. Tolls CJ: Gynecologic cancer associated with pregnancy. *Sem in Oncol* 1989; 16: 417–24.
2. Atar E, Dgani R, Shoham (Schwartz) Z, Borenstein R: Ovarian cancer during pregnancy. *Harefuah* 1990; 119: 146–8.
3. Beral V, Frazer P, Chilvers C: Does pregnancy protect against ovarian cancer? *Lancet* 1978; i: 1083–7.
4. Beischer NA, Buttery BW, Fortune DW *et al*: Growth and malignancy of ovarian tumors in pregnancy. *Aust NZ J Obstet Gynecol* 1971; 11: 208–20.
5. Chung A, Birenbaum SJ: Ovarian cancer complicating pregnancy. *Obstet Gynecol* 1973; 41: 211–14.
6. Novak ER, Lambrov CO, Woodruff JO: Ovarian tumors in pregnancy. *Obstet Gynecol* 1975; 46: 401–6.
7. Dgani R, Shoham (Schwartz) Z, Atad *et al*: Ovarian carcinoma during pregnancy: a study of 23 cases in Israel between the years 1960 and 1984. *Gynecol Oncol* 1989; 33: 326–31.
8. Jubb ED: Primary ovarian carcinoma in pregnancy. *Am J Obstet Gynecol* 1963; 85: 345–54.
9. Mitchell DG, Mintz MC, Spritzer CE *et al*: Adnexal masses: MR imaging observations at 1.5 T, with US and CT correlation. *Radiology* 1987; 162: 319–24.
10. Kier R, McCarthy SM, Scoutt LM *et al*: Pelvic masses in pregnancy: MR imaging. *Radiology* 1990; 176: 709–13.
11. Matsuyama T, Tsukamoto N, Mastukuma K *et al*: Malignant ovarian tumors associated with pregnancy: report of six cases. *Int J Gynecol Obstet* 1989; 28: 61–6.
12. DiSaia PJ, Creasman WT: *Clinical Gynecologic Oncology.* 1984, p. 277, Wiley, New York.
13. Brodsky JB, Cohen EN, Brown BW *et al*: Surgery during pregnancy and fetal outcome. *Am J Obstet Gynecol* 1980; 138: 1165–67.
14. Hill LM, Johnson CE, Lee RA: Ovarian surgery in pregnancy. *Am J Obstet Gynecol* 1975; 122: 565–9.
15. Hess LW, Peaceman A, O'Brien WF *et al*: Adnexal mass occurring with intrauterine pregnancy: Report of 54 patients requiring laparotomy for definitive management. *Am J Obstet Gynecol* 1988; 158: 1029–34.
16. Buttery BW, Beischer NA, Fortune DW *et al*: Ovarian tumors in pregnancy. *Med J Aust* 1973; 1: 345–9.
17. Ashkenazy M, Kessler B, Czernobilsky B *et al*: Ovarian tumors in pregnancy. *Int J Gynecol Obstet* 1988; 27: 79–83.

13
Malignant melanoma and pregnancy

M. RAVID, M. LISHNER, D. ZEMLICKIS
AND G. KOREN

To the students of human malignancies, malignant melanoma (MM) presents a continuous challenge. Depending on specific circumstances, this tumor may be aggressive and rapidly lethal, while in a different set-up it may be dormant for many years. It is easily resectable at its early stages and practically incurable when advanced. Above all, it is preventable by such simple measures as careful periodic examination of the skin, especially in high-risk patients and avoidance of excessive exposure to solar irradiation.

Melanoma originates from individual melanocytes, pigment cells present in the epidermis and dermis, in about two-thirds of the cases and from pre-existing cutaneous naevi in one-third[1,2]. The incidence of melanoma has increased substantially over the past decades[3,4]. It is estimated that approximately 29 000 new cases are diagnosed annually in the United States resulting is 6000 deaths. If this trend continues, the individual lifetime risk for this tumor will be 1%. The average age at presentation is 45 years[3] and in some countries the incidence in women is almost double that in men[4–6]. It has been noted, however, that from the time of diagnosis women have a longer survival than men[7–9].

Although men present with metastatic disease more often than women, the latter survive longer also with the same extent of disease[10–13]. In stage 1 disease the most important prognostic factor is the tumor thickness at the time of resection, with five-year survival declining from 96–99% in lesions thinner than 0.76 mm to a corresponding figure of only 44–47% for lesions thicker than 4 mm[3]. Generally women present with thinner lesions than men[10]. However, women have a higher survival for each thickness level. In contrast, Weidner[14] who examined the eight-year survival in a large group of clinical stage 1 patients having 1.5 mm or thicker lesions found no statistically significant survival advantage of women when compared for site of lesion. In this study women had a better overall survival after four years but the curves of men and women were almost parallel after eight years. It has been postulated that melanoma might be androgen dependent since the tumor doubling time was found to be somewhat shorter in men than in women[15]. Others, however, found estrogen and progesterone receptors on specimens of malignant melanoma[16,17].

These findings form some of the background to the questions of the behavior of melanoma in pregnancy and the possible effect of pregnancy and other hormonal interventions on the incidence and on the rate of recurrence of this tumor.

Of women with melanoma, 30–35% are of child-bearing age[3,18]. Furthermore, with the increase in age of marriage and in number of older women having children, a larger proportion of women, who have had melanoma successfully resected, are still in their reproductive period and may become pregnant. In view of the potential hormonal potentiating effect on the rate of growth of melanoma, the question of whether a subsequent pregnancy may alter the outlook becomes critical. Until 1989 only some 200 cases of melanoma in pregnancy were documented and reported[19]. The articles comprised mainly case reports or small series and there was no stratification for the thickness of the primary lesion or site which are, no doubt, the dominant determinants of prognosis[3,20,21]. Three large series[22–24] published between 1989–91 together reported on 246 women with stage 1 malignant melanoma diagnosed during pregnancy. These series deepened our knowledge about the influence of pregnancy on the diagnosis and course of melanoma. They were all well controlled for primary lesion thickness and site.

Among the patients followed by the World Health Organization melanoma programme[22], there were 92 diagnosed during pregnancy, 85 who were treated before pregnancy, 68 between pregnancies, and 143 after they had completed all pregnancies. Survival curves of the four groups showed the best overall survival and disease-free survival among the patients who were diagnosed and treated before their pregnancies and the worst survival among those patients in whom melanoma was diagnosed during pregnancy. The mean tumor thickness, however, was 2.38 mm in the pregnant women as compared to 1.49 mm in those diagnosed before they became pregnant. When log rank adjustment was made for tumor thickness, there was no difference in survival between the various groups. Wong *et al*[23] investigated 66 women in whom melanoma was diagnosed while they were pregnant. Survival of these women was not different from a group of 619 nonpregnant women with similar thickness of the primary tumor (1.24 mm in the pregnant women versus 1.28 mm in the nonpregnant). In these groups all patients, pregnant and nonpregnant with tumor thickness greater than 0.65 mm had regional lymph node dissection. Slingluff *et al*[24] reported 88 stage 1 patients who were pregnant at the time of diagnosis. In this series, the tumor thickness was greater in the pregnant than in the nonpregnant patients. Multivariate analysis, stratifying for tumor site and thickness, showed no difference in survival between the pregnant and nonpregnant groups. The unequivocal conclusion of these three large studies would therefore be that, once the thickness of the primary lesion is controlled for, there is no difference in survival between patients with melanoma diagnosed during, before or after pregnancy. In a later publication of his results and a summary of recent literature, Slingfull[25] also concludes that pregnancy in itself was not a risk factor for patient mortality. However, from the clinician's point of view when actual survival, disease-free period, and time to metastatic spread are considered, the available data show that pregnant women are diagnosed at a later stage and thus show a worse prognosis. The median disease-free intervals for pregnant and nonpregnant women were 5.8 and 11.9 years, respectively. At 10 years, lymph node metastases developed in 48% of the pregnant patients and only in 26% of the nonpregnant patients ($p = 0.008$)[25].

Two reviews published in 1993[26,27] also summarize that stratification for tumor site and thickness abolishes the difference in disease free interval and overall survival between pregnant and nonpregnant patients. However, they also stress that, actually, women with melanoma diagnosed during pregnancy tend to have thicker tumors, shorter disease-free interval and lower 10-year survival rate than nonpregnant matched controls. They also stress that there is no no conclusive evidence that therapeutic abortion improves the cure rates. A summary of the German experience based on the registry of the German Dermatological Society[28] revealed that 1% of female melanoma patients were pregnant, and 40% were found when in their premenopausal period. They also found no statistical differences in survival rates between the pregnant and nonpregnant patients. A similar conclusion was put forward also in a recent American review[29].

In summary, it seems that the controlled studies of recent years have produced a reasonable consensus.

It is possible to conclude that pregnancy does not alter the prognosis of women with melanoma whether the woman is pregnant at the time of diagnosis or becomes so after successful treatment.

Advice to women who wish to become pregnant after treatment of stage 1 disease should be based on primary tumor thickness, body site and evidence of tumor cells in vascular channels. Women with primary melanoma of less than 1.5 mm thickness have very good survival. The survival is compromised when the tumors are thicker[22]. For stage 2 disease, it has been shown that 83% of women present with metastatic disease within 2 years of the resection of the primary tumor[22]. It is therefore wise to avoid pregnancy during the first 3 years subsequent to the surgical treatment of melanoma. Later on, there seems to be no increased risk for melanoma associated with subsequent pregnancies[22,28]. There is no role of therapeutic abortion for the indication of maternal tumor regression.

Several studies over the years, have claimed that pregnancy may have a favorable effect on survival of patients who subsequently develop malignant melanoma[7,29,30]. The actual figures in those studies, however, were not impressively significant. Hersey *et al*[29] reported the five-year survival of 77% and 68% for women with and without previous pregnancies. Show *et al*[7] found the corresponding ratios to be 81.6% and 73.8% respectively. Elwood and Coldman[30], however, failed to demonstrate any difference in five-year survival between previously pregnant and nonpregnant women, while Lederman and Sobel[31] found a better nine-year survival for the never pregnant group (87%) than the parous patients (83%). This ratio persisted also when only women above 50 were considered. All these studies were retrospective and share the common flaw of inaccurate clinical data, especially tumor site and thickness.

Malignant melanoma accounts for about 8% of malignancies during pregnancy. However, it comprises about one-third of all tumors with transplacental spread to the fetus[32]. It is of particular interest that, in some cases of fetal metastasis of melanoma, the tumor subsequently regressed and the infants survived. It was speculated that the regression was due to homograft rejection. Also, three rare cases of primary fetal melanoma were also published[33]. Generally, it is safe to say that transplacental spread of tumors in general and melanoma in particular is uncommon. This risk does not justify therapeutic abortion.

It was previously claimed that, during pregnancy, there is a threefold higher incidence of melanoma as compared to nonpregnant women[19]. This, and the hyperpigmentation of the nipples, the linear alba and other areas of the skin during pregnancy were ascribed to increased secretion of melanocyte stimulating hormone and other growth factors[18,19,34,35]. The color changes which take place in pregnancy may also account, in part, for the somewhat delayed diagnosis of melanoma in pregnant women[22]. Later reports, however, failed to demonstrate any increase in the incidence of melanoma in pregnant women[32].

Likewise, contrary to several anecdotal reports[13,15] there is no well-documented evidence of regression of melanoma upon termination of pregnancy. Also the results of all hormonal manipulations (e.g., hypophysectomy, antiestrogens, androgens, etc.) were disappointing[36]. Snell and Bischitz[37] showed that estrogen and progesterone cause an increase in melanocyte count and in intra- and extracellular melanin content. Prolonged administration of estrogens in the form of oral contraceptive preparations was shown to increase the number of estrogen receptors in cells of pigmented nevi[38]. The number of estrogen and progesterone receptors on melanocytes or on cells of melanoma specimens is relatively small as compared to known hormone-sensitive tumors (e.g., breast, prostate)[39,40]. These observations prompted clinical observational studies that aimed to find an association between the use of oral contraceptives and the incidence of malignant melanoma. As so often observed by longitudinal watchers of medical research, early reports found a clear-cut increase in the incidence of melanoma in users of oral contraceptives[41-43]; however, later more carefully planned studies failed to show such an effect. Several case control studies[44,45] and an epidemiological study which compared the overall incidence of melanoma in women of child-bearing age to men[46] concluded that prolonged use of oral contraception was not associated with a significant added risk of malignant melanoma. Based on seven large studies, the relative risk for the development of melanoma for prolonged users of oral contraceptives compared to nonusers was 1.12 (95 confidence interval 0.94–1.33)[45].

The early observations of increased incidence of malignant melanoma in users of oral contraceptives could be explained, in part, by the subsequent observation that users of oral contraceptives tended to enjoy more sunlight exposure than nonusers[47].

Our own experience in the Princess Margaret Hospital includes 21 cases of melanoma and pregnancy identified in the 30 years analyzed in our study. One woman had two pregnancies, both of which fit in the time frame of the study, resulting in a total of 22 pregnancies in 21 women. In our series, the survival experience over a 30 year period is 70%. At the time of the study, five of the cases had died of melanoma, whereas the remaining 16 either lived or died of other causes. The mean age of pregnant women with melanoma was 27–5.4 years at diagnosis. The median age was 27 years (range 18 to 37 years).

Of the 22 pregnancies, four were terminated by therapeutic abortions and there were 18 deliveries. Of the 18 deliveries, there were 17 live births and one anencephalic stillbirth with spina bifida. This mother's only

Table 13.1. *Comparison of fetal outcome in mothers with melanoma with that of a matched control group*

	n	PMH	n	MR
Gestational age (wks)	13	39.54 ± 2.67	13	40.08 ± 1.55^{a}
Number of preterm births (< 37 wks)	13	1	13	0
Birth weight (g)	9	3036 ± 597	9	3392 ± 371^{b}
Delivery method	15		13	
Spontaneous		13		10
C/S		2		3
Malformations	15	1 anencephalic stillbirth	13	None

[a]p = 0.53.
[b]p = 0.15.

treatment during pregnancy was excision of the malignant mole at 28 weeks' gestation. Two of the deliveries were by cesarean section; one of these was to allow initiation of therapy for melanoma, whereas the remaining case was for noncancer related obstetrical difficulties.

We were able to obtain 12 obstetrical records from the delivering hospitals and one autopsy report. The remaining delivery records could not be obtained because some charts did not indicate the delivering hospital, or the delivering hospital had destroyed the old birth records. In some cases the delivering hospital refused to release confidential documents without the patient's signature. A summary of the available information regarding fetal outcome is presented in Table 13.1. There was a trend towards lower birth weight, as compared to their matched controls, which did not reach statistical significance mobably due to the small sample size. There was no statistical difference in mean gestational age (p = 0.53), suggesting that the differences in birth weight were due to intrauterine growth retardation secondary to the melanoma, its therapies or complications.

A detailed therapeutic approach to malignant melanoma is beyond the scope of this chapter. Early detection and treatment, especially in pregnant women who tend to have hyperpigmentation, is highly important. Suspicious lesions should be biopsied and the diagnosis established by pathologic examination. Surgery is the only effective curative treatment for this disease. The thickness and margins of the resection are determined by the lesion's thickness and site[18]. The role of lymph node dissection is controversial and this issue should be clarified by ongoing studies. Metastatic melanoma is very resistant to chemo and radiotherapy and, in the pregnant woman, maternal salvage should be balanced against fetal risks. Immunotherapy remains experimental in all patients and especially in pregnant women.

In summary, the clinical course of malignant melanoma in pregnancy has been the subject of a long term controversy. The current evidence, however, strongly suggests that it is not different from the clinical course in nonpregnant women. Likewise, oral contraception or estrogen replacement therapy are not associated with an increased risk to develop melanoma. Available data do not permit one to support continuous use of any form of hormone therapy when melanoma is diagnosed and in the first two to three years of follow-up. Since over 85% of the recurrences take place within this time limit, it is prudent also to avoid subsequent pregnancy during this period. There is, however, no direct evidence that such pregnancies are associated with an increased risk of early recurrence.

The tendency of hyperpigmentation in pregnancy calls for very careful examination of the skin especially in high-risk patients (fair skin, blue eyes, a history of sunburn before age 10, freckles). Early diagnosis and biopsy of localized disease enables surgical excision of the primary lesion and an excellent prognosis. As in men and nonpregnant women, the most important prognostic factor for stage 1 melanoma in pregnancy is the thickness of the primary lesion. There is no evidence to support a therapeutic abortion following excision of stage 1 disease. In advanced disease, termination of pregnancy may become necessary in order to enable uninterrupted combined chemotherapy. Transplacental spread is very uncommon, nevertheless a careful examination of the fetus by ultrasound should be undertaken in each case.

References

1. Briel HA, Das Gupta TK: Natural history of cutaneous malignant melanoma. *World J Surg* 1979; 3: 255–8.
2. Seigler HF, Fetter BF: Current management of melanoma. *Ann Surg* 1977; 186: 1–12.
3. Balch CM, Soong S-J, Shaw HM, Milton GM: An analysis of prognostic factors in 4000 patients with cutaneous melanoma. In *Cutaneous Melanoma*. (Balch CM, Milton GW, ed.), 1985, p. 328, J.B. Lippincott, Philadelphia.
4. MacKie RM, Smyth JF, Soutar DS *et al*: Malignant melanoma in Scotland 1979–1983. *Lancet* 1985; ii: 859–62.
5. Adam YG, Efron G: Cutaneous malignant melanoma; current views on pathogenesis, diagnosis and surgical management. *Surgery* 1983; 93: 481–94.
6. Lee JAH, Storer BH: Excess of malignant melanoma in women in the British Isles. *Lancet* 1980; ii: 1337–9.
7. Shaw HM, Mieton GW, Farago G *et al*: Endocrine influences on survival from malignant melanoma. *Cancer* 1978; 42: 667–9.

8. Blois MS, Sagebiel RW, Abarbanel RM *et al*: Malignant melanoma of the skin. The association of tumor depth and type, and patient sex, age and site with survival. *Cancer* 1983; 52: 1330–41.

9. Lee YN: Better prognosis of many cancers in females. A phenomenon not explained by study of steroid receptors. *J Surg Oncol* 1984; 25: 255–62.

10. Shaw HM, McGovern VJ, Milton GW *et al*: Histologic features of tumors and the female superiority in survival from malignant melanoma. *Cancer* 1980; 45: 1604–1608.

11. Shaw HM, McGovern VJ, Milton GW *et al:* The female superiority in clinical stage II cutaneous malignant melanoma. *Cancer* 1982; 49: 1941–4.

12. Griffel M: Survival of cutaneous malignant melanoma patients at University of Iowa hospitals. *Cancer* 1981; 47: 176–83.

13. Rampen F: Malignant melanoma: sex differences in survival after evidence of distant metastasis. *Br J Cancer* 1980; 42: 52–7.

14. Weidner F: Eight year survival in malignant melanoma related to sex and tumor location. *Dermatologica* 1981; 162: 51–60.

15. Rampen FH, Mulder JH: Malignant melanoma: an androgen-dependent tumor? *Lancet*, 1980; 1: 562–4.

16. Fisher RI, Neifeld JP, Lippman ME: Oestrogen receptors in human malignant melanoma. *Lancet* 1976; ii: 337–8.

17. Creagan ET, Ingle JN, Woods JE *et al*: Estrogen in patients with malignant melanoma. *Cancer* 1980; 46: 1785–6.

18. Wong DJ, Strassner HT: Melanoma in pregnancy. *Clin Obstet Gynecol* 1990; 33: 782–9.

19. Fiora B, Hauven D: Malignant melanoma, sex hormones and pregnancy. *Harefuah* 1989; 117: 314–17.

20. Balch CM, Murad TM, Soong SJ, Ingalls AL, Richards PC, Maddox WA: Tumor thickness as a guide to surgical management of clinical stage 1 melanoma patients. *Cancer* 1979; 43: 883–8.

21. Day CL, Mihm ML, Lew RA, Kopf AW, Sober AJ, Fitzpatrick TB: Cutaneous malignant melanoma: prognostic guidelines for physicians and patients. *CA* 1982; 32: 113.

22. MacKie RM, Bufalino R, Morabito A, Sutherland C, Cascinelli N: Lack of effect of pregnancy on outcome of melanoma. *Lancet* 1991; 337: 653–5.

23. Wong JH, Sterns EE, Kopald KH *et al*: Prognostic significance of pregnancy in stage 1 melanoma. *Arch Surg* 1989; 124: 1227–31.

24. Slingluff CL, Reintgen DS, Vollmer RT, Seigler HF: Malignant melanoma arising during pregnancy: a study of 100 patients. *Ann Surg* 1990; 211: 552–9.

25. Slingluff CL, Seigler HF: Malignant melanoma and pregnancy. *Ann Plast Surg* 1992; 28: 95–9.

26. Driscoll MS, Jorgensen GCM, Kels GJM: Does pregnancy influence the prognosis of malignant melanoma? *J Acad Dermatol* 1993; 29: 619–30.

27. Kjems E, Krag C: Melanoma and pregnancy. A review. *Acta Oncol* 1993; 32: 371–8.

28. Garbe C: Pregnancy, hormone preparations and malignant melanoma. *Hautarzt* 1993; 44: 347–52.

29. Hersey P, Morgan G, Stone DE *et al*: Previous pregnancy as a protective factor against death from melanoma. *Lancet* 1977; i: 451–2.

30. Elwood JM, Colman AJ: Previous pregnancy and melanoma prognosis. *Lancet* 1978; ii: 1000–1.

31. Lederman JS, Sober AJ: Effect of prior pregnancy on melanoma survival.

Arch Dermatol 1985; 121: 716 (editorial).

32. Colbourn DS, Nathanson L, Belilos E: Pregnancy and malignant melanoma. *Semin Oncol* 1989; 16: 377–87.

33. Campbell WA, Storlazzi E, Vintzileos AM *et al*: Fetal malignant melanoma: ultrasound presentation and review of the literature. *Obstet Gynecol* 1987; 70: 434–9.

34. Sutherland CM, Wittliff JL, Fuchs A, Mabie WC: The effect of hormone levels and receptors in malignant melanoma. *J Surg Oncol* 1983; 22: 191–2.

35. Byrd BF, McGAnity WJ: The effect of pregnancy on the clinical course of malignant melanoma. *South Med J* 1954; 47: 196–200.

36. Nathanson L, Julkarni GA: Endocrine influences on the natural history of human malignant melanoma. In *Basic and Clinical Aspects of Malignant Melanoma*. (Nathanson L, ed.) 1987, pp. 131–139, Boston, Nijhoff.

37. Snell RS, Bischitz PG: The effect of large doses of estrogen and estrogen and progesterone on melanin pigmentation. *J Invest Dermatol* 1960; 35: 73–83.

38. Schwartz BK, Zashin SJ, Spencer SK *et al*: Pregnancy and hormonal influences on malignant melanoma. *J Dermatol Surg Oncol* 1987; 13: 276–81.

39. Fisher RI, Neifeld JP, Lippman ME: Estrogen receptors in human malignant melanoma. *Lancet* 1976; ii: 337–8.

40. Chaudhuri PK, Wlaker MJ, Briele HA *et al*: Incidence of estrogen receptors in benign nevi and human malignant melanoma. *JAMA* 1980; 244: 791–3.

41. Beral V, Ramcharan S, Faris R: Malignant melanoma and oral contraceptive use among women in California. *Br J Cancer* 1977; 36: 804–9.

42. Lerner AB, Nordlund JJ, Kirkwood JM: Effects of oral contraceptives and pregnancy on melanoma. *New Engl J Med* 1979; 301: 47.

43. Holly EA, Weiss NS, Liff JM: Cutaneous melanoma in relation to exogenous hormones and reproductive factors. *JNCI* 1983; 70: 827–31.

44. Adam SA, Sheaves JK, Wright NH *et al*: A case control study of the possible association between oral contraceptives and malignant melanoma. *Br J Cancer* 1981; 44: 45–50.

45. Holman CD, Armstrong BK, Heenan PJ: Cutaneous malignant melanoma in women: exogenous sex hormones and reproductive factors. *Br J Cancer* 1984; 50: 673–80.

46. Danforth DN, Russell N, McBride CM: Hormonal status of patients with primary malignant melanoma: a review of 313 cases. *South Med J* 1982; 75: 661–4.

47. Ramcharn S, Pellegrin FA, Ray RM *et al*: The Walnut Creek oral contraceptive study. An interim report. *J Reprod Med* 1980; 25: 346–72.

14

Leukemia during pregnancy

M. LISHNER AND M. RAVID

The information regarding leukemia complicating pregnancy is very limited. Since there is no systematic registration of leukemia in pregnancy, the existing knowledge is based mainly on retrospective analyses or case reports. These reports tend to describe unusual or successful cases. Thus, review articles of the published experience may have perpetuated a reporting bias. Leukemia occurring during pregnancy is very rare with an estimated incidence of one per 100000 pregnancies annually[1,2]. This figure is about 3.5 times lower than the incidence of leukemia in the general population in the Western world. This lower incidence may be explained by the fact that most acute lymphatic leukemias occur in childhood, while most acute myeloid leukemias occur in late adulthood, thus relatively sparing the child-bearing years[3]. Chronic myeloid leukemia is the main chronic leukemia during pregnancy, since chronic lymphocytic leukemia is founded mainly in the elderly.

It had been estimated that, during pregnancy, acute leukemias are more frequent than chronic and that myeloid leukemias are detected twice as often as lymphatic leukemias[4]. The appearance of leukemia during the first trimester of pregnancy is least common, and may be explained by the use of therapeutic abortion in patients diagnosed in this trimester[1,4].

The survival of pregnant and nonpregnant leukemic women has improved with the availability of modern chemotherapy and supportive care. Remission rates of 70–75% and median survival time of 6–12 months are currently reported for pregnant women[1,2]. These figures are not different from those achieved in young nonpregnant women with acute leukemia. No prospective studies comparing nonpregnant and pregnant women with acute leukemia are available, but there are no data to suggest that pregnancy has an impact on the course and prognosis of acute leukemia.

The leukemia can affect pregnancy and the fetus. Intrauterine growth retardation has been reported even in mothers not treated with chemotherapy[1,5]. In addition, preterm labor, both induced and spontaneous, is common in acute leukemia[1]. These expected complications occur even more frequently when the mothers are treated with chemotherapy[6].

The effect of antileukemic therapy on pregnancy is detailed in Chapter 17. In summary, short term toxicity on the fetus includes bone marrow depression[7,8]. However, this is usually mild and short lived. Teratogenic effects of combination chemotherapy in the first trimester, with agents used to treat acute leukemia (antimetabolites, vinca alkaloids and anthracyclines), appear at an estimated rate of 10%[9]. Administration of chemotherapy in later trimesters does not seem to carry teratogenic risk[10]. Reynoso *et al*[7] studied long-term effects in children whose mothers received chemotherapy during pregnancy. After follow-up ranging between 1 and 17 years, the children had normal growth and sexual and intellectual development. There is only one report of a malignant tumor that developed in one of twins whose mother was treated during pregnancy for acute leukemia[7,11].

Management decisions in pregnant women with acute leukemia are extremely complicated and should be resolved in collaboration between the physicians, the patient and her family. It is generally believed that pregnant women should be treated as nonpregnant women[1,4]. Therapeutic abortion should be considered in early gestation[1] and if the woman decides to proceed with pregnancy, teratogenic drugs such as methotrexate should be avoided[10]. Standard antileukemic treatment can be safely administered during the second and third trimester[4,10]. Delivery should be accomplished when fetal survival can be ensured and the mother is in complete remission.

Chronic myeloid leukemia (CML) during pregnancy is rare. Since the disease has an initial chronic phase, it is usually managed conservatively during pregnancy, while aggressive approach (i.e., bone marrow transplantation) may be considered after delivery. Single case reports describe successful treatment modalities of CML during pregnancy and include leukapheresis[12,13], hydroxyurea[14] and interferon[15,16]. It does not appear that pregnancy adversely affects the course of CML.

In summary, the scarce available data suggest that the approach to leukemia during pregnancy should not differ from the approach to nonpregnant patients. There are, however, several exceptions to this approach:

- When the leukemia is diagnosed before or during the first trimester, the option of termination of pregnancy should be discussed with the family.

- If pregnancy is continued, chemotherapy should be postponed until after the completion of embryogenesis (12 weeks of gestation).
- The mother and fetus should be closely followed by a tertiary high-risk obstetric unit, where the team should be led by the oncologist and perinatologist.
- Delivery should be performed at a time which ensures optimal balance between fetal maturity and maternal well-being.

References

1. Catanzarite VA, Ferguson JE: Acute leukemia and pregnancy: a review of management and outcome. *Obstet Gynecol Surv* 1984; 39: 663–78.
2. Haas VA: Pregnancy in association with newly diagnosed cancer: a population-based epidemiologic assessment. *Int J Cancer* 1984; 34: 229–35.
3. National Cancer Institute: *Third National Cancer Survey: Incidence Data* (Culter SJ, Young JL Jr, eds.) 1975, p. 102, National Cancer Institute Monograph No. 41, Government Printing Office, Washington DC.
4. Caliguiri MA, Mayer RA: Pregnancy and leukemia. *Sem Oncol* 1989; 16: 388–96.
5. Nicholson HO: Leukemia and pregnancy: a report of 5 cases and discussion of management. *J Obstet Gynecol Br Commonw* 1968; 75: 517–20.
6. Felin J, Ivarez S, Ordonez A, Gracia-Paredes ML, Gonazalez-Baron M, Montero JM: Acute leukemia and pregnancy. *Cancer* 1988; 61: 580–4.
7. Reynoso EE, Shepherd FA, Messner HA *et al*: Acute leukemia during pregnancy. The Toronto Leukemia Study Group experience with long-term follow-up of children exposed *in utero* to chemotherapeutic agents. *J Clin Oncol* 1987; 5: 1098–2106.
8. Colbert N, Najman A, Gorim NL *et al*: Leucemie argue un cours de la grossesse, évolution favorable de la gestation chez deux mâlades traitées par chimiotherapie. *Presse Med* 1980; 9: 175–8.
9. Koren G, Weiner L, Lishner M, Zemlickis D, Finegan J: Cancer in pregnancy: identification of unanswered questions on maternal and fetal risks. *Obstet Gynecol Surv* 1990; 45: 509–14.
10. Lishner M, Koren G: *Fetal Risks of Cancer Chemotherapy in Pregnancy.* (Nisker JA, Allen HH, Sutcliffe SB, eds.), Futura Publications, New York, in press.
11. Zemlickis D, Lishner M, Erlich R, Koren G: Teratogenicity and carcinogenicity in a twin exposed *in utero* to cyclophosphamide. *Teratogenesis, Carcinogen Mutagen.* 1993; 13: 139–43.
12. Bazarbashi MS, Smith MR, Karanes C, Zielinski I, Bishop CR: Successful management of Ph chromosome positive chronic myelogenous leukemia with leukapheresis during pregnancy. *Am J Hematol* 1991; 38: 235–7.
13. Nolan TE, Ross WB, Caldwell C: Chronic granulocytic leukemia in pregnancy. A case report. *J Reprod Med* 1988; 33: 661–3.
14. Patel M, Dukes IA, Hull JC: Use of hydroxyurea in chronic myeloid leukemia during pregnancy: a case report. *Am J Obstet Gynecol* 1991; 163: 565–6.
15. Crump M, Wang XH, Sermer M, Keating A: Successful pregnancy and delivery during alpha interferon treatment for chronic myeloid leukemia

(letter). *Am J Hematol* 1992; 40: 238–9.
16. Baer MR, Ozer H, Foon KA: Interferon-alpha therapy during pregnancy in chronic myelogenous leukemia and hair cell leukemia. *Br J Haematol* 1992; 81: 167–9.

15
Thyroid cancer and pregnancy

I. B. ROSEN

Introduction

The thyroid gland undergoes changes during and following pregnancy which have been repeatedly described[1-4]. These widely reported changes are essential for the understanding of the various thyroid affectations that are special for the pregnant patient. The commonest cancer of the thyroid gland, i.e. the well-differentiated variety, is frequent in females of fertile age. It is still undecided whether thyroid cancer diagnosed during pregnancy represents as a coincidental or a cause-related phenomenon. The effect of pregnancy on the behaviour of such a cancer is of some importance.

Changes in thyroid status with pregnancy

In pregnancy there is a 40% increase in maternal blood volume which contributes to an increased glomerular filtration rate and increased renal iodide clearance which produces in essence a decline in maternal serum iodide which reaches its maximum effect in the second trimester. Such a deficit is coupled with increased thyroid iodine clearance. Radioiodine thyroid uptake is increased during pregnancy and is consistent with some histological studies which have shown thyroid follicular cell hypertrophy and hyperplasia. Goiter formation can develop as a compensatory mechanism in iodine deficient areas. Fetal iodine stores reflect the state of maternal iodine deficiency[1-3].

Thyroxine binding globulin (TBG) increases more than twofold during pregnancy, with its maximum level being detected at the end of the first trimester. This increase is due to estrogen secretion by the placenta and increased serum TBG due to production of variants which are cleared from the circulation more slowly than normal forms of TBG. Thyroxine binding prealbumin declines slightly or does not change at all during pregnancy and hypoalbuminemia may develop but this affects little the overall binding or distribution of T-4 amongst several proteins[1-3].

Stimulation of thyroid hormone secretion includes the in-pregnancy thyroid stimulating hormone (TSH) as well as the much weaker human chorionic gonadotropin (HCG), although estimates of its potency in this regard are variable. HCG reaches its peak at the end of the first trimester and may show a small secondary peak with the approach of term but this is of minimal proportion[1-3].

The placenta is impermeable to maternal TSH but is presumably permeable to thyrotropin releasing hormone (TRH). On the basis of animal experimentation, it is felt that maternal thyroid hormones reach the fetus early in pregnancy before the developing fetal thyroid can function. High concentrations of T-3 in the maternal circulation do not inhibit high serum TSH concentrations in hypothyroid neonates. Some authors have noted that serum levels of T-4 and T-3 increase during pregnancy as does TBG but T-4 and T-3 rises were not commensurate with the elevation in TBG. Analysis of free hormone states during the three trimesters reveals a substantial decrease in free T-4 and T-3 as pregnancy progresses, and a relative hypothyroxinemia is felt to occur in one-third of pregnant patients, although TSH does not elevate into the hypothyroid range.

Although some authors question the clinical significance of these changes[3], it is widely agreed that thyroid function tests at six months postpartum are similar to those seen in a nonpregnant control group.

While the increase in serum T-4 and T-3 concentrations is viewed as reflecting the increase in serum TBG, it is important to determine free hormone levels. Serum TSH concentrations may decline during the first trimester presumably due to a small increase in thyroid secretion by HCG. Serum thyroglobulin concentrations increase during the first trimester of pregnancy with 50% of women having an above normal value.

It has been generally agreed that increase in size of the thyroid gland is common during pregnancy. It is of interest to note that 71% of pregnant patients in Scotland with a low iodine state showed goiter formation whereas only 37% of a nonpregnant control group were similarly affected[2]. In North American studies, it has been felt that there is no substantial difference of goiter or thyroid enlargement between control groups of pregnant and nonpregnant women implying that thyroid enlargement in pregnant women represents a pathological condition. When sonography has been used in evaluation, it showed a 20 to 30% increase in thyroid volume during pregnancy. Where thyroid supplementation is utilized,

Table 15.1. *Changes in thyroid status during pregnancy[1–3]*

Thyroid antibodies		Decrease
CD 4 + /Cd 8 + T cells		Decrease
Thyroid enlargement	(I_2 ↓)	Marked
	(I_2 ↑)	Minimal
TBG		Increase
T-3		Increase
T-4		Increase
FT-3		Decrease (minor?)
FT-4		Decrease (minor?)
Thyroglobulin		Increase
TSH		No change
HCG		Increase
T-3 RU		Decrease
BMR		Increase

ultrasonography has indicated that there is a significant reduction of thyroid gland enlargement. Iodine-treated women exhibit a 15% increase in thyroid gland size as opposed to a 35% increase in untreated controls. Furthermore, in a small number of patients affected by thyroid gland enlargement, the abnormal size persisted for one year postpartum[2].

Changes in the maternal immune system do occur during pregnancy. A progressive decrease in CD4 plus T cells has been described as was a progressive decline in CD 4+/CD 8 + T cells throughout pregnancy. These immunological changes are felt to be critical in the acceptance of the fetal allograft. This dampened immunological system does ameliorate the course of autoimmune diseases. There is a further decrease in thyroid antibodies, most particularly antithyroglobulin and antithyroidoperoxidase as well as TSH receptor immunoglobulins throughout pregnancy. Women have been shown to develop a marked decline in thyroid antibody titres during pregnancy, regardless of the development of postpartum thyroiditis or not[2]. Elevated CD 4+/CD 8 + ratio are seen in women who develop postpartum thyroid dysfunction (Table 15.1).

Thyroid cancer in pregnancy

It has been suggested that pregnancy poses little problem in thyroid cancer, with only few cancer patients treated during pregnancy. Cunningham[5] cited the work of Roswell and Winship who found no evidence that pregnancy and thyroid cancer were related; in 38 pregnant patients treated for thyroid carcinoma, the course of cancer was unremarkable, resulting in a disease-free state which was not reactivated by subsequent pregnancies.

In 1985, Rosen[6] described 20 patients with thyroid nodular disease who were hyperthyroid. There was a 43% rate of cancer in 16 nontoxic thyroid nodules with three instances of metastatic nodal disease. Two patients underwent mid-trimester surgery without ill effect. In 1986, Rosen[7] reported on 30 patients with thyroid neoplasia, one-quarter of whom showed significant growth during pregnancy. Twenty-six operations were done with 24 in the postpartum period. There was a 43% incidence of cancer and 37% incidence of adenoma for a total neoplasia rate of 80%. There was no significant morbidity from surgery. One woman treated conservatively with thyroid suppression to await postpartum surgery experienced stillbirth at term. Review of these cases suggested a pregnancy-associated trophic influence on thyroid cancer behavior.

McTiernan[8] described 389 women with thyroid cancer who had been interviewed regarding medical and reproductive histories and who were compared to a random sample of controls. Women who had a history of breast cancer were three times more likely to develop thyroid cancer. Infertility, late age at first full-term pregnancy, early age at menarche, abortion and miscarriage did not appear to influence the occurrence of thyroid cancer. Increased body weight was found to be an additional risk factor.

Franceschi[9] studied 165 women with thyroid cancer and 214 controls to investigate the role of reproductive and hormonal factors as etiological factors. Late age at menarche, menstrual irregularity and late age at first birth significantly correlated with development of thyroid cancer both in premenopausal and postmenopausal women. Parity was inconsistently related to disease status whereas voluntary abortions and miscarriages were completely unrelated. Increased risk was associated with age, menopause beyond 50 years of age and the use of oral contraceptives in premenopausal women. The actual mechanism of endocrine implication appeared unresolved.

Yoshimura[10] presented work on the mechanism of thyroid stimulation by human chorionic gonadotropin in the sera of normal pregnant women, and his results suggested that thyrotropic activity of HCG in sera of normal pregnant women is at least in part mediated by TSH receptors.

Akslen[11] noted that in 64000 Norwegian women there were 124 cases of thyroid cancer between 1961 and 1989. No strong associations with reproductive factors or parity were noted. A long reproductive period was related to increased risk of papillary cancer with a decreased risk of follicular cancer. Risk of thyroid cancer was slightly increased amongst women in the occupational category of ship officers and crew.

Casara[12] described 70 female patients who had been treated with high doses of I-131 for thyroid cancer and who had undergone subsequent pregnancy. He concluded that the previous administration of high dose I-131 did not appear to be a valid reason for dissuading young female patients from considering pregnancy, although he cautioned about the need to avoid pregnancy for a year after radioiodine.

Levi[13] conducted a study in 91 women with thyroid cancer and 306 controls in order to investigate the role of reproductive and hormonal factors in the etiology of this malignancy. There was a questionable increase in cancer risk with increasing number of full-term pregnancies and spontaneous abortions. Most other reproductive, menstrual and hormonal factors did not seem to affect the risk of thyroid cancer.

Wingren[14] reviewed 104 patients in Sweden and observed that for women less than 50 years of age there was an increased risk for thyroid cancer in pregnancy occurring soon after puberty, as well as with increasing number of pregnancies. Multiparity seemed to potentiate the effect of previous radiographic examination.

Kobayashi[15] reported two cases of papillary cancer during pregnancy which grew rapidly in the first trimester suggesting a tumorgenic influence of HCG.

In 1994 at the Triological Society meeting, Mestman's group[16] reported a review of 23 patients with thyroid nodules detected during pregnancy. Incidence of malignancy in their experience was 39%, and four patients had undergone surgery during pregnancy and seven patients were operated on in the postpartum period. There was no incidence of fetal morbidity or mortality.

Herzon[17] reported on all cases of well-differentiated cancer in patients age 18 to 46 retrieved from the New Mexico Tumor Registry. Followup ranged from 6 months to 20 years. Four hundred and sixty-five women between 18 and 46 comprised the nonpregnant group and 22 the pregnant study group. They noted that, while thyroid cancer is presumed to occur as 1% of all cancers, it represented 83% of head and neck cancer cases in women between 18 and 46 in their experience. Six patients received surgery during pregnancy and I-131 was delayed until the postpartum period of time. There were no statistical differences in the courses of cancer between pregnant and nonpregnant patients. The authors were mindful of the possibility of increased fetal risk that had been suggested in older literature but felt that there was no improvement in survival rate with surgical treatment during the gestational period and that delay until the postpartum period was advisable.

Thyroid cancer management

Papillary follicular carcinoma which makes up about 80% of all thyroid malignancies is generally viewed as unaggressive in nature and compatible with prolonged survival and cure. Mazzaferri[18] has recently analyzed his experience and noted a mortality rate of 8% and a recurrence rate of 30%. Recurrences were most frequent at the extremes of age, namely patients younger than 20 and older than 59 years of age. Cancer mortality was lowest in patients younger than 40 years of age but increased with each subsequent decade of life and only 2% of patients younger than 40 died. Other important predictors of recurrence and death included tumor size in excess of 2.5 cm, regional lymph node metastases, local tumor invasion, three or more multicentric sites of thyroid malignancy with increasing tumor stage. Patients who underwent treatment within a year showed a 4% mortality rate as opposed to 10% who were treated after a year's duration. A near-total thyroidectomy appears to offer the patient a slightly better chance for recurrence and mortality avoidance. Furthermore, the use of adjuvant radioiodine appears to offer the patient survival advantage as compared to external radiation. Patients treated with radioiodine showed a recurrence rate of 20% as compared to 41% in patients who had not received I-131. No patient receiving I-131, according to Mazzaferri, has died of this disease.

In the post-treatment phase, patients should be assessed periodically for recurrent disease by clinical and radiological methods. Thyroglobulin status is particularly helpful in the patient with total thyroidectomy and normal antithyroglobulin titres. Scintiscanning techniques with Sestamibi for detection of recurrence are currently being assessed. Management of recurrent disease may require further surgery, radioiodine ablation or external radiation.

Conclusions

Thyroid cancer affects women particularly during their childbearing years. Despite this, there has been a paucity of reports of the pregnant patient with thyroid cancer. The effects of pregnancy on the course and biology of well-differentiated thyroid cancer have not been documented probably because of the very low-grade activity of this malignancy. The very comparable survival periods and apparent innocuousness of behavior of well-differentiated cancer in both pregnant and nonpregnant patients has cultivated an attitude of *laissez faire* and a general feeling of treatment

Table 15.2. *Algorithm of manangement of pregnant thyroid nodule*

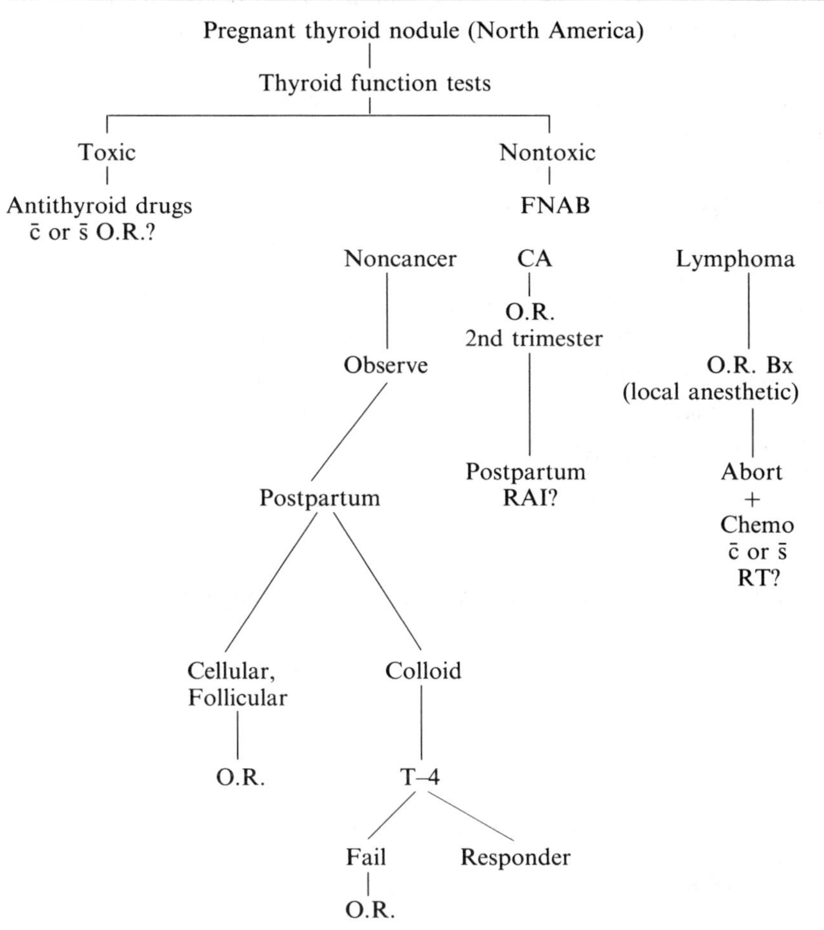

delay until after parturition. Nevertheless, observations have been made[12] of an accelerated growth pattern, and even a predisposition for metastasis in pregnant patients. Although the numbers are small and no statistical proof of definite aggravation of malignant behavior by pregnancy is presently possible, these reports serve to remind us that there is at least a cause for unease. The patient who is pregnant may pose particular problems for management since there has to be an avoidance of radioiodine, chemotherapeutic drugs, external radiation, and even thyroid scintiscanning. It is generally agreed that surgery during the middle trimester of pregnancy avoids the problems of first trimester teratogenesis and last trimester premature delivery. It is our feeling that thyroid cancer which is usually established by fine needle aspiration biopsy is still best treated on an expeditious basis to avoid the infrequent aggressive course which can theoretically be lethal for the euthyroid patient.

Since surgery in the middle trimester appears safe for both mother and fetus[14–16], it would appear best to manage thyroid cancer during that time if feasible. Table 15.2 presents an algorithm of management of thyroid cancer during pregnancy. The concerns for adverse effects that may affect the pregnant patient and her unborn baby should be taken into account, and delay of treatment should be considered in the face of a nonmalignant FNAB until the postpartum period of time. At all times the family's feelings regarding the pregnancy must be factored into cancer management policy on an individualized basis. Increased awareness and further inquiry will undoubtedly enhance our knowledge of the role and management principles of thyroid cancer recognized during pregnancy.

Acknowledgements

The author acknowledges the very considerable support of the endo-crinological expertise of Dr Paul G. Walfish, and assistance in paper preparation by Dr Dan Farine and Mrs Margaret Allen.

References

1. Emerson C: Thyroid disease during and after pregnancy. In *Thyroid*, (Braverman L, Utiger R, eds.) 1991, pp. 1263–128, JB Lippincott Company, New York.
2. Stagnero-Green A: Pregnancy in thyroid disease. *Immunol. Allergy Clin. N Am.*, 1994; 14: 865–78.
3. Inzucchi S, Comite F, Burrow G: Graves' disease and pregnancy. *End. Pr.* 1995; 1: 186–92.
4. Donnigan W: Cancer and pregnancy. *Cancer*, 1983; 33: 194–214.
5. Cunningham M, Slaughter D: Surgical treatment of disease of the thyroid gland in pregnancy. *SGO* 1970; 131: 486–8.
6. Rosen I, Walfish P, Nikore V: Pregnancy in surgical thyroid disease. *Surgery* 1985; 98: 1135–40.
7. Rosen I, Walfish P: Pregnancy as a disposing factor in thyroid neoplasia. *Arch Surg* 1986; 121: 1287–90.
8. McTiernan A, Weiss N, Daling J: Incidence of thyroid cancer in women in relation to known or suspected risk factors for breast cancer. *Can Res* 1987; 47: 292–5.
9. Franceschi S, Facina A, Talamini R *et al*: The influence of reproductive and hormonal factors on thyroid cancer in women. *Review d'Epidemelogie et de Sante Publique*, 1990; 38: 27–34.

10. Yoshimura M, Nishikawa M, Yoshikawa N *et al*: Mechanism of thyroid stimulation by human chorionic gonadotrophin in sera of normal pregnant women. *Acta Endocrinol*, 1991; 124: 173–8.
11. Akslen IA, Nilssen S, Kvale G: Reproductive factors and risk of thyroid cancer. *Br J Cancer*, 1992; 65: 772–4.
12. Casara D, Rubello D, Saladini G *et al*: Pregnancy after high therapeutic doses of iodine-131 in differentiated thyroid cancer. *Eur J Nucl Med* 1993; 20(3): 192–4.
13. Levi F, Franceschi S, Gulie C *et al*: Female thyroid cancer. *Oncology* 1993; 50: 309–15.
14. Wingren G, Hatschek T, Axelson O: Determinance of papillary cancer of the thyroid. *Am J Epidemiol* 1993; 138: 482–91.
15. Kobayashi K, Tanaka Y, Ishiguro S *et al*: Rapidly growing thyroid carcinoma during pregnancy. *J Surg Oncol* 1994; 55: 61–4.
16. Doherty C, Shindo M, Rice D *et al*: Management of thyroid nodules during pregnancy. *Laryngoscope* 1995; 105: 251–5.
17. Herzon F, Morris D, Siegel M *et al*: Coexistent thyroid cancer in pregnancy. *Arch Autolaryngol Head Neck Surg* 1994; 120: 1191–3.
18. Mazzaferri E, Jhiang S: Long term impact in initial surgical and medical therapy on papillary and follicular thyroid cancer. *Am J Med* 1994; 97: 418–28.

Part III

Fetal effects of cancer and its treatment

16
Prenatal irradiation and cancer

YEDIDIA BENTUR

Ionizing radiation includes gamma rays, X-rays and particulate radiation. The first two are short wavelength electromagnetic waves composed of high-energy photons and lower-energy photons, respectively.

Particulate radiation is generated from the spontaneous disintegration of radioactive compounds, resulting in emission of alpha particles (helium nuclei), beta particles (electrons) and other forms of energy.

X-rays and gamma rays penetrate tissues deeply, but generate ions sparsely along their path. Therefore, they are considered as having low linear energy transfer (LET) as opposed to particulate radiation.

Ionizing radiation can be expressed in units of exposure (roentgen-R), its absorbance into biologic tissue (rad, gray-Gy) and as biological effectiveness of absorbed radiation (roentgen equivalent man-rem, sievert-Sv). For radiation in soft tissue, rad and rem are often used interchangeably. One hundred rad or rem are 1 Gy or 1 Sv, respectively.

Ionizing radiation can damage biological cells by two mechanisms. The first involves addition of sufficient energy to incite electron shells to free an electron from its atomic orbit, thereby producing charged or ionized biological molecules. The second mechanism involves radiolysis of water to form reactive compounds (e.g., OH^-, H^+, H_2O_2) which can attack and disrupt neighboring molecules.

The insult from a single, random modification of a cell component (e.g., DNA) is termed a *stochastic effect* and it may still allow the cell to proliferate. Therefore, dose–response curves for effects such as mutagenesis and carcinogenesis may not include a threshold below which no adverse effects occur. It is assumed that this effect may be associated even with very low doses of ionizing radiation and there is great uncertainty as to how to best predict unavoidable injurious effects from such an exposure. On the other hand, a *nonstochastic effect* is produced by numerous and/or repeated damage. Its dose–response curve is expected to show a tissue specific threshold above which damage is detectable. This type of injury may also involve various compensatory and repair mechanisms which may explain increased tolerance of tissues to fractionated radiation dose. Radiation-induced malformations are probably a nonstochastic effect[1].

Humans could be exposed to several sources of low- or high-level ionizing radiation: (i) background radiation consisting of low-level radiation coming from soil and rocks (terrestrial), building materials, air, sun and stars; (ii) occupational (laboratories, radiology institutes, nuclear power plants, etc.); (iii) medical: radiodiagnosis and radiotherapy; (iv) disasters and accidents (e.g., the atomic bombing of Hiroshima and Nagasaki, Chernobyl, Nevada test site). It is the high-level exposures in disasters and certain occupations (e.g., uranium miners) that brought the most striking evidence of the carcinogenic effects of ionizing radiation and stimulated serious studies.

However, most human exposure to ionizing radiation is associated with its medical use, especially radiodiagnostic procedures which involve low-level radiation. In 1980, 80 million fertile women and men were exposed to X-ray procedures in the USA; 30000 were women in their early pregnancies and the numbers continue to grow[2].

Epidemiological studies established the potential of ionizing radiation to induce leukemia and solid tumors in children and adults[3,4]. Irradiation of infants for thymic hyperplasia, for example, is clearly associated with the subsequent development of carcinoma of the thyroid[5]. The Life Span Study of the atomic bomb survivors showed that leukemia is the most striking cancer, reaching a peak 6–7 years after the bombing. The risk of leukemia was greater during the early period post-exposure, as the subjects' age was younger at the time of bombing[6]. Relative risk for death from cancer other than leukemia was also higher as age was younger at time of exposure[6,7]. In addition, a dose-related increase in cancer was observed for some digestive organs[6]. Boice suggested that as much as 3–5% of all cancers might be attributed to all sources of radiation, including medical, occupational and environmental exposures[8].

The following discussion will focus on the evidence for the potential of prenatal radiation to cause cancer in childhood and later on in life.

Surprisingly, irradiation of mice with doses between 30 and 100 rad at various stages of pregnancy did not induce a statistically significant increase in the incidence of tumors in the offspring[9–11]. Einhorn suggested that, although organogenesis involves pronounced cell proliferation and differentiation, it is highly resistant to carcinogenesis. A possible explanation is the existence of highly active regulators influencing development which may control cancer[12].

However, epidemiological studies are not always in agreement with these notions. As happens many times, they are subjected to methodological limitations such as selection bias, recall bias, small cohort, inadequate ascertainment of data, inadequate control for other risk factors, postnatal exposure to radiation, different radiation sources and techniques, different methods of radiation dose estimation, different gestational ages at exposure and insufficient long-term follow-up.

Controversy begins as one looks at data for preconception exposure to radiation. Graham reported an identical increased risk of leukemia for offspring of mothers who had radiodiagnostic procedures shortly before or after conception[13]. Children who were conceived after the atomic bombing and were born to proximally exposed survivors ($<$ 2000 m from hypocenter) from May 1946 to December 1958 (bombs were dropped in August 1945) did not have an increase in cancer risk. This holds also for the high-dose exposed group. Of these children, 90% have been exposed to $\geq$ 0.01 Sv, as estimated by the revised and more accurate Dosimetry System 1986 (DS86). This study has to be continued since follow-ups included those who were younger than 20 years of age between 1946 and 1982[14]. Gardner *et al* found raised relative risks for leukemia and non-Hodgkin's lymphoma among children born to fathers employed at the Sellafield nuclear plant, particularly those with high recorded radiation doses before the child's conception[15]. Another study from Dounreay nuclear installation could not come to the same conclusions[16]. As part of the Oxford Survey of Childhood Cancer (OSCC), estimates were made for paternal exposure to human-made external ionizing radiation (as judged from job histories) in the six months before conception of 15279 children dying from cancer. Assessments were also made for potential exposure to unsealed source of radionuclides. Relative risk assessed by multiple logistic regression was close to unity for most points of exposure to external ionizing radiation, but it was 2.87 (95% CI 1.15–7.13) for adionuclide exposure[17].

It is hard to draw conclusions as to the carcinogenic potential of preconception exposure to radiation because study parameters are not always comparable: maternal vs paternal or both parents' exposure, cancer deaths vs incident cases, high and acute radiation dose vs low and/or fractionated dose and different radiation sources.

Several studies, many of them based on the OSCC, suggested that *in utero* exposure to radiodiagnostic procedures may cause leukemia and possible other cancers in humans[13,18–27]. The increase in the risk for leukemia in these studies ranged from 1.3 to about 3.0. Risk of cancer was greatest when exposure was during the first trimester[19]. Excess cancer risk was not found in black population[25]. Many of the radiodiagnostic procedures involved pelvimetry and it was suggested that irradiation received by fetal gonads frequently exceeded 2.5 rad[20]. Others could not demonstrate an increase in leukemia after such procedures[28,29]. Stewart discusses some methodological problems which could have been responsible for low leukemia incidence found in some studies, especially prospective ones. An important limitation is the existence of very few radiogenic leukemias among the cases which are diagnosed before 5 years of age and a sizeable number among the cases diagnosed between 5 and 10 years of age[18]. Brent, when reviewing these studies, pointed out a number of parameters which were suggested to be associated with leukemia: upper respiratory infections, strong family history of allergy, history of abortion or stillbirth, maternal smoking and heavier birth weight[30]. It is unclear to what extent these parameters contribute to post-*utero* radiation leukemia, if at all. Could it be that the examinations attracted preleukemic children, but not caused the disease, or the radiation had aggravated a disease process? Or, maybe stillbirth or neonatal death prevented recognition of an early leukemia death[18]?

Reanalysis of the data of the OSCC in 1988 again confirmed the association between obstetric X-raying and childhood cancer, including the increased risk in the first trimester[31]. Interestingly, Mole showed from the OSCC data that excess cancer deaths decreased suddenly for births in and after 1958. During 1957 and early 1958, fetal radiation dose reductions were achieved in Britain by reducing the rising rate of obstetric radiography, especially pelvimetry. In the 1970s, the rate of X-raying increased again and so did cancer risk, but insignificantly. For example, odds ratio for 1953–1957 and 1958–1961 were 1.62 (90% CI 1.4–1.87) and 1.23 (90% CI 1.05–1.44), respectively[32].

In order to overcome selection bias, studies were conducted in twins exposed prenatally to X-ray to determine twin status and their position, rather than of maternal or fetal medical condition which could predispose to cancer. A study on 32000 twins born in Connecticut (only 31 had cancers) showed a relative risk of 2.4 (95% CI 1.0–5.9) for leukemia or other cancer, after birth weight was adjusted. The relative risk for solid tumors was greater than that for leukemia (3.2 vs 1.6, respectively). Twins who were 10–14 years of age at diagnosis had an increased risk. The two latter findings were not in accordance with other studies. Children whose mothers had experienced previous pregnancy loss had higher relative risk compared to those whose mothers had not (7.8 vs 1.4, respectively)[32]. A larger Swedish case-control twin study which included 95 cases of childhood cancer showed similar results. The relative risks for all cancers, leukemia and CNS tumors in children of women who had abdominal X-ray was 1.4, 1.7 and 1.5, respectively. The relative risk for second trimester exposure was 8.0 and 1.1 for third trimester. There was no apparent confounding by mother's age, drug use, obstetric complications, previous miscarriage, social class or length of pregnancy[33,34].

Original estimates of cancer deaths after *in utero* exposure to radiodiagnostic procedures ranged between 40 and 50%[27,35]. Stewart and Kneale derived a 10-year mortality estimate of 57 deaths per million children exposed per mGy (95% CI 30–80)[19]. The United Nations Scientific Committee on the Effects of Atomic Radiation (UNSCEAR) estimate was 29[36]. Bithell and Stiller's more recent death estimate is 20.9 (95% CI 12.5–31.8), probably reflecting reduced use of obstetric radiography and improved survival of children with tumors. They went on and calculated cancer incidence and found it to be 175 extra cases per million irradiated fetuses with 1 mGy in the first 15 years of life[31]. The UNSCEAR earlier estimate was 240 cases per million per rad[36]. Mole found a risk coefficient for irradiation in the first trimester for childhood cancer deaths at ages 0–15 years of 4–5×10^{-4} per cGy fetal whole body dose (95% CI 0.8–95×10^{-4} per cGy). It is the same for cancer incidence and mortality[32]. In comparison to all of this, a 2-rad dose delivered to an adult population would not demonstrate a perceptible incidence of leukemia, even for large population groups[30].

Early studies of the *in utero*-exposed atomic bomb survivors could not demonstrate an increase in cancer mortality and incidence of leukemia in childhood, although these patients received considerably high doses of radiation[37–40]. Later on, Yoshimoto *et al* observed 18 incident cases of cancers among these survivors in the years 1950–1984. Five of the cases were in the zero-dose group. Two of these patients had childhood cancer (liver cancer and Wilm's tumor) in the first 14 years of life. Both were exposed to 0.30 Gy or more. All other cases developed cancer in adulthood. Cancer risk appeared to increase significantly as maternal uterine dose increased. Compared to the 0 Gy group, the ≥ 0.30 Gy group developed cancer earlier and the incidence continued to increase. The crude cumulative incidence rate in this high-dose group during the 40 years after the bombing was 3.9 higher than in the 0 Gy group. These authors estimated the relative risk of cancer at 1 Gy to be 3.77 (95% CI 1.14–13.48). For the entire ≥ 0.01 Gy group, the average excess risk per 10^4 person–year–gray is 6.57 (95% CI

0.47–14.49) and the estimated attributable risk is 40.9% (2.9–90.2%). No significant differences were found in the risk of radiation-related cancer associated with exposure in different gestational periods. They suggested that individuals prenatally exposed to the atomic bomb are more susceptible to radiation-induced cancers than exposed adults because they have not reached the major cancer prone age. However, the number of cases observed by Yoshimoto *et al* is small and further follow-up studies are needed[14,41,42].

The apparently low rate of childhood cancer after prenatal exposure to the atomic bomb radiation observed in the early studies of survivors has often been regarded as conflicting with the higher rate found in prenatal medical radiology. Although the recent findings of Yoshimoto *et al* may suggest a greater risk for radiogenic cancers in the prenatally exposed atomic bomb survivors than has been previously thought, there are more reasons to suggest that the conflict is not serious.

More than 20 years ago, Stewart suggested an expanding cell population and survival of the host to be essential prerequisites for clone formation and tumor development[19]. Ionizing radiation can induce cell transformation, but high doses will also inactivate these cells and prevent their multiplication. Thus, the observed frequency of induced malignant disease after exposure to high radiation doses in the inactivation range could be less than the frequency expected from the induction or transformation process[43]. Much of the population of bomb survivors irradiated *in utero* came from the highest dose group and cell inactivation is expected[32]. Moreover, most of the Japanese information about irradiation *in utero* comes from Hiroshima where the proportion of the maternal dose due to neutrons was much higher than at Nagasaki. Neutrons are more effective per rad in inactivating cells. Although they are more carcinogenic than gamma rays, their inactivating action may markedly reduce the expected yield of malignant disease[43]. Yoshimoto *et al* pointed out also that, for those alive with cancer, ascertainment of tumor registries before 1960 is incomplete and could not cover those who migrated from a registry's reporting area. Migration was greater in younger individuals and in Nagasaki. Thus, they suggested that absolute risk of cancer incidence may be underestimated by 15–20%[41]. Finally, Mole suggested that the lower risk in bomb survivors exposed *in utero* is not incompatible since its confidence intervals are wide and well within the confidence intervals for the risk he derived for diagnostic X-rays[32].

Summary

Intense studies suggest that humans appear less sensitive to the genetic effects of radiation than previously thought and emphasize the importance of radiation-induced somatic changes[8,14,44]. The 'cancer mutation' probably marks the start of a process which begins by having a high probability of being interrupted, and ends by having a high probability of causing disease[18]. Despite numerous studies which correlate childhood leukemia with prenatal radiation, there is still uncertainty if it plays a causative or associative role[8,30]. Further follow-up of survivors is needed as it is suggested that they may be at increased risk of cancer in adult life[14]. A significantly raised cancer rate after low-dose diagnostic X-raying supports the hypothesis that carcinogenesis by ionizing radiation has no threshold[8,32]. Smith, from the International Commission on Radiological Protection, concluded that *in utero* irradiation is not considered likely significantly to influence the lifetime risk of a person living to old age who is irradiated throughout life[45].

When looking at the estimates of 40–50% increased risk after prenatal radiation, one should also consider the risk of leukemia in other populations and the meaning of this figure. The risk for leukemia up to the age of 10 years in US white children less than 15 years ago was 1 : 2800, in children exposed *in utero* to pelvimetry 1 : 2000, and in siblings of leukemic children 1 : 720[30]. If one were inclined to recommend therapeutic abortion on these grounds, one would perform abortions in 1999 exposed nonleukemic subjects for every leukemic subject "saved"[30]. It is not the common medical practice to recommend an abortion for a sibling of a leukemic child whose risk is much greater than the irradiated fetus. The biologic knowledge is only one facet to be considered, and the "spontaneous risks" of pregnancy should be recognized.

References

1. Bentur Y: Ionizing and nonionizing radiation in pregnancy. In: *Maternal–Fetal Toxicology* (Koren G, ed.) 2nd ed. 1994 pp. 515–572. Marcel-Dekker Inc., New York.
2. Mossman KL: Medical radiodiagnosis and pregnancy: evaluation of options when pregnancy status is uncertain. *Health Phys* 1985; 48: 297–301.
3. Advisory Committee on the Biological Effects of Ionizing Radiation. *The Effects on Populations of Exposure to Low Levels of Ionizing Radiation*. 1980, National Research Council, National Academy of Sciences, National Academy Press, Washington DC.
4. Polhemus D, Koch R: Leukemia and medical irradiation. *Pediatrics* 1959; 23: 453–61.

5. Favus MJ, Schneider AB, Stachura ME *et al*: Thyroid cancer occurring as a late consequence of head-and-neck irradiation. *New Engl J Med* 1976; 294: 1019–25.

6. Shimizu Y, Schull WJ, Kato H: Cancer risk among atomic bomb survivors: The RERF Life Span Study. *JAMA* 1990; 264: 601–4.

7. Kato H, Schull WJ: Studies of the mortality of A-bomb survivors 9. Mortality, 1950–78, part I: cancer mortality. *Radiat Res* 1982; 90: 395–432.

8. Boice Jr JD: Studies of atomic bomb survivors. Understanding radiation effects. *JAMA* 1990; 264: 622–3.

9. Rugh R, Duhamel L, Skaredoff L: Relation of embryonic and fetal X-irradiation to life-time average weights and tumor incidence in mice. *Proc Soc Biol Med* 1966; 121: 714–18.

10. Brent RL: The response of the $9\frac{1}{2}$ day old rat embryo to variations in dose rate of 150 R X-irradiation. *Radiat Res* 1971; 45: 127–36.

11. Brent RL, Bolden BT. The indirect effect of irradiation on embryonic development. The lethal effects of maternal irradiation on the first day of gestation in the rat. *Proc Soc Exp Biol Med* 1967; 125: 709–12.

12. Einhorn L: Can prenatal irradiation protect the embryo from tumor development? *Acta Oncol* 1991; 30: 291–9.

13. Graham S, Levin MI, Lilienfeld AM, Schuman LM, Gibson R, Dowd JE, Hempelmann L: Preconception, intrauterine and postnatal irradiation as related to leukemia. *Natl Cancer Inst Monograph* 1966; 19: 347–71.

14. Yoshimoto Y: Cancer risk among children of atomic bomb survivors: a review of RERF epidemiologic studies. *JAMA* 1990; 264: 596–600.

15. Gardner MJ, Snee MP, Hall AJ, Powell CA, Downes S, Terrell JD: Results of case-control study of leukemia and lymphoma among young people near Sellafield nuclear plant in West Cumbria. *Br Med J* 1990; 300: 423–9.

16. Urquhart JD, Black RJ, Muirhead MJ, Sharp L, Maxwell M, Eden OB, Jones DA: Case-control study of leukemia and non-Hodgkin's lymphoma in children in Caithness near the Dounreay nuclear installation. *Br Med J* 1991; 302: 687–92.

17. Sorahan T, Roberts PJ: Childhood cancer and paternal exposure to ionizing radiation: preliminary findings from the Oxford Survey of Childhood Cancers. *Am J Ind Med* 1993; 23: 343–54.

18. Stewart A: The carcinogenic effects of low-level radiation: A reappraisal of epidemiologists' methods and observations. *Health Phys* 1973; 24: 223–40.

19. Stewart A, Kneale GW: Radiation dose effects in relation to obstetric X-rays and childhood cancers. *Lancet* 1970; 1: 1185–8.

20. Stewart A, Webb J, Giles G, Hewitt D: Malignant disease in childhood and diagnostic irradiation *in utero*. *Lancet* 1956; 2: 447.

21. Stewart A, Webb J, Hewitt D: A survey of childhood malignancies. *Br Med J* 1958; 1: 1495–508.

22. Lilienfeld AM: Epidemiological studies of the leukemic effects of radiation. *Yale J Biol Med* 1966; 39: 143–64.

23. Ager EA, Schuman LM, Wallace HM *et al*: An epidemiological study of childhood leukemia. *J Chron Dis* 1965; 18: 113–32.

24. Ford D, Patterson T: Fetal exposure to diagnostic X-rays and leukemia and other malignant diseases in childhood. *J Natl Cancer Inst* 1959; 22: 1093–104.

25. Diamond EL, Schmerler H, Lilienfeld AM: The relationship of intrauterine radiation to subsequent mortality and development of leukemia in children. A prospective study. *Am J Epidemiol* 1973; 97: 283–313.

26. Kneale GW, Stewart AM: Prenatal X-rays and cancers: Further tests of data from the Oxford Survey of Childhood Cancers. *Health Phys* 1986; 3: 369–76.
27. MacMahon B: Prenatal X-ray exposure and childhood cancer. *J Natl Cancer Inst* 1962; 28: 1173–91.
28. Tabuchi A, Nakagawa S, Hirai T *et al*: Fetal hazards due to X-ray diagnosis during pregnancy. *Hiroshima J Med Sci* 1967; 16: 49–66.
29. Court Brown WM, Doll R, Bradford Hill A: Incidence of leukemia after exposure to diagnostic radiation *in utero*. *Br Med J* 1960; (5212): 1539–45.
30. Brent RL: The effect of embryonic and fetal exposure to X-ray, microwave and ultrasound: counselling the pregnant and nonpregnant patient about these risks. *Semin Oncol* 1989; 16: 347–68.
31. Bithell JF, Stiller CA: A new calculation of the carcinogenic risk of obstetric X-raying. *Stat Med* 1988; 7: 857–64.
32. Mole RH: Childhood cancer after prenatal exposure to diagnostic X-ray examination in Britain. *Br J Cancer* 1990; 62: 152–68.
33. Harvey EB, Boice Jr JD, Honeyman M, Flannery JT: Prenatal X-ray exposure and childhood cancer in twins. *New Eng J Med* 1985; 312: 541–5.
34. Rodvall Y, Pershagen G, Hrubec Z, Ahlbom A, Pederson NL, Boice JD: Prenatal X-ray exposure and childhood cancer in Swedish twins. *Int J Cancer* 1990; 46: 362–5.
35. Bithell JF, Stewart AM: Prenatal irradiation and childhood malignancy: a review of British data from the Oxford Survey. *Br J Cancer* 1975; 31: 271–87.
36. UNSCEAR: *Ionizing Radiation: Levels and Effects. Vol II: Effects.* 1972, United Nations, New York.
37. Joblon S, Kato H: Childhood cancer in relation to prenatal exposure to atomic-bomb radiation. *Lancet* 1970; ii: 1000–3.
38. Kato H: Mortality in children exosed to the A-bombs while *in utero*, 1945–69. *Am J Epidemiol* 1971; 93: 435–42.
39. Burrow GN, Hamilton HB, Hrubec Z: Study of adolescents exposed *in utero* to the atomic bomb, Nagasaki, Japan. I. General aspects: clinical and laboratory data. *Yale J Biol Med* 1964; 36: 430–44.
40. Ishimaru T, Ishimaru M, Mikami M: Leukemia incidence among individuals exposed *in utero*, children of A-bomb survivors, and their controls; Hiroshima and Nagasaki, 1945–79. (RERF Tech Rep 11–81) Hiroshima: Radiation Effects Research Foundation, 1981.
41. Yoshimoto Y, Kato H, Schull WJ: Risk of cancer among children exposed *in utero* to A-bomb radiations, 1950–84. *Lancet* 1988; ii: 665–9.
42. Yoshimoto Y, Kato H, Schull WJ: A review of forty-five years study of Hiroshima and Nagasaki atomic bomb survivors: cancer risk among *in utero* survivors. *J Radiat Res (Tokyo)* 1991; 32 (suppl): 231–8.
43. Mole RH: Antenatal irradiation and childhood cancer: causation or coincidence? *Br J Cancer* 1974; 30: 199–208.
44. Neel JV, Schull WJ, Awa AA *et al*: The children of parents exposed to atomic bombs: estimates of the genetic doubling dose of radiation for humans. *Am J Hum Genet* 1990; 46: 1053–72.
45. Smith H: The detrimental health effects of ionizing radiation. *Nucl Med Commun* 1992; 13: 4–10.

17

Review of fetal effects of cancer chemotherapeutic agents

D. ZEMLICKIS, M. LISHNER AND G. KOREN

Cancer chemotherapeutic drugs are among the most potent teratogens known[1]. Since they are administered at maximum tolerated dose, the risk of teratogenesis is great. In fact, Nicholson, in his seminal review of chemotherapy usage in pregnancy, estimated that the risk of malformations is 10% when cytotoxic drugs are administered in the first trimester in contrast to the 1–3% baseline[2,3].

Currently, there is very little information on the effects of chemotherapeutic treatment on the fetus; available information is based primarily on case reports. This paucity of data probably reflects a lack of experience in treating pregnant women and a tendency amongst oncologists to avoid chemotherapeutic treatment during pregnancy.

Most cases reported deal mainly with the presence or absence of morphological adverse effects. Commonly, neonates are described as "normal" without qualifying the term. For example, hematological values of neonates exposed to chemotherapeutic drugs are rarely reported. Occasionally details of laboratory results and physical exams are given, but long term follow-ups are seldom performed. Even basic details such as birth weight are often omitted.

Several chemotherapeutic drugs are teratogenic and mutagenic in laboratory animals; however, animal results cannot be directly extrapolated to humans[4]. In animals, the fetus is most sensitive to malformations during the middle third of pregnancy[5]. In humans this has not been shown. The risk of fetal malformation following chemotherapy in the second or third trimester is not greater than normal[2,6], but in the second and third trimester the risk of intrauterine growth retardation and premature labor is higher than normal[7].

Differences between animal and human outcomes may be related to differences in dosage, gestation period, drug metabolism, and the time cycle

168

of fetal development[5]. Therefore, animal data can only *suggest* a potential danger to the human fetus.

The cell cycle

Chemotherapeutic drugs are classified by their mechanism of action. Different classes of drugs operate at different points in the cell's life cycle. The cell cycle has four active stages (G_1, S, G_2, M) and an inactive or resting stage (G_0)[8]. A cell spends most of its time in the G1 phase which prepares the cell for DNA synthesis. The S phase is the phase of chromosomal doubling. In the G_2 phase the mitotic apparatus is formed to prepare for the M phase. Mitosis occurs in the M phase where the cell divides into two cells[9].

Alkylating agents

Alkylating agents are cell cycle nonspecific and operate during most parts of the cell cycles. They form cross-linkages with DNA thus inhibiting cell division and normal biological activity. In addition, they alkylate proteins and may attack macromolecules independent of DNA synthesis, making them valuable in treating resting (G_0) cells[9].

Nitrogen mustard

In animal studies, nitrogen mustard has been found to be a teratogen in all species tested. In a review, Schardein (1993) summarized digital anomalies and hydrocephalus in mice; cleft palate, central nervous system, and chromosomal abnormalities were found in rats.

In humans, Barber[4] reported on three women exposed to nitrogen mustard during the first four months of pregnancy. All three delivered normal infants. Nicholson[2] reviewed eight other pregnancies where nitrogen mustard was used in three patients during the first trimester. One pregnancy was terminated, three resulted in spontaneous abortion, and four live babies were delivered with no abnormalities. Garrett[10] reported on a child delivered at 24 weeks of gestation with abnormalities of both feet and the right tibia, as well as a cerebral hemorrhage. The mother had received nitrogen mustard, vinblastine, and procarbazine during the first trimester. The use of combination chemotherapy in this case makes it impossible to implicate nitrogen mustard alone. The risk of malformation due to nitrogen mustard would appear to be approximately $1:3$[11].

Cyclophosphamide

Cyclophosphamide is metabolized in the liver by cytochrome P-450 to 4-hydroxycyclophosphamide (4-OHCP) which exists in equilibrium with aldophosphamide. Aldophosphamide undergoes spontaneous degradation catalyzed intracellularly by protein, cellular enzymes, and bases to form phosphoramide mustard and acrolein. 4-OHCP and phosphamide mustard are cytotoxic *in vivo* and *in vitro*, but only the latter functions at physiological pH. Therefore, phosphoramide mustard is considered to be the ultimate alkylating agent. 4-OHCP and aldophosphamide can be oxidized to form inactive products by the enzyme aldehyde dehydrogenase, producing 4-ketocyclophosphamide and carboxyphosphamide, respectively[12].

There is some dispute in the literature whether phosphoramide mustard or acrolein is the ultimate cause of teratogenicity[13–15]. Hales[13] injected into the amniotic fluid of pregnant rats phosphoramide mustard and acrolein. The malformations found in the fetuses produced by acrolein included forelimb and hindlimb defects, cleft palate, hydrocephaly, edema, and open eyes. In contrast, phosphoramide mustard produced only hydrocephaly, forelimb and hindlimb defects.

In humans, administration of cyclophosphamide in the first trimester in a patient with Hodgkin's disease resulted in a male child with four toes on each foot, flattened nasal ridge, and bilateral inguinal hernia sacs[16]. Toledo *et al*[17] reported on a 28 year-old pregnant woman with Hodgkin's disease with cyclophosphamide and radiation (estimated dose to uterus was 5 to 25 rads) in the first trimester. At $25\frac{1}{2}$ weeks' gestation, hypertonic saline was injected into the amniotic sac and 48 hours later she spontaneously passed a dead male fetus. The fetus was missing all of its toes and an autopsy showed a single left coronary artery.

Several authors have reported on a unique case of daily cyclophosphamide and intermittent prednisone maintenance treatment throughout gestation[18,19]. The mother delivered a male twin with multiple congenital anomalies who was diagnosed with papillary thyroid cancer at 11 years of age and stage 3 neuroblastoma at 14 years of age. The female twin was unaffected and has exhibited normal development to date. The estimated risk of malformation with cyclophosphamide is 1 : 6[11].

Chlorambucil

Chlorambucil has been found to induce cleft palate, limb defects, and hernias in mice, as well as digit and tail anomalies, cleft palate, and CNS defects in rats[11].

A 27 year-old woman with Hodgkin's disease was treated daily with 6 mg of chlorambucil throughout the first trimester. Therapeutic abortion was performed and a fetal biopsy revealed an absent kidney and ureter on the left side[20]. Barber[4] reports no significant increase in fetal damage from the use of chlorambucil. The estimated risk of malformation with this drug is 1 : 2[11].

Busulfan

In pregnant rats who received intraperitoneal doses of busulfan, gonadal hypoplasia and stunted growth have been reported[21].

Intrauterine growth retardation has been reported in a baby after first trimester exposure to busulfan[22]. Infants of normal weight have also been reported after first trimester exposure[23].

Diamond *et al*[24] reported on a mother who received busulfan throughout the pregnancy. 6-mercaptopurine was instituted at 36 weeks' gestation. The woman delivered a female infant at 39 weeks' gestation with bilateral corneal opacities, cleft palate, and bilateral microphthalmia. The baby did not maintain her body weight and died ten weeks after birth.

Abramovici *et al*[25] report on a six-week old embryo therapeutically aborted from its 39 year-old mother. The mother was treated with busulfan prior to pregnancy and during the first trimester. On examination, the embryo was found to have myeloschisis, a neural tube defect. The authors suggest that maternal age may have been a factor. The estimated risk of malformation with this drug is 1 : 9[11].

Cisplatin

Cisplatin exerts its antineoplastic effect by cross-linking DNA and, therefore, may be considered an alkylating agent[8]. Platinum thymine blue (related to *cis*-platinum) produced eye defects, hydrocephalus, and embryonic death in rats[26].

In a case report by Jacobs *et al*[27] a woman was treated with cisplatin at ten weeks of gestation. At 12 weeks' gestation, a hysterectomy was performed. Fetal autospy showed no abnormalities.

We have encountered a case of cisplatin used at $29\frac{1}{2}$ weeks gestation of pregnancy in a patient with ovarian cancer. Twelve days after chemotherapy, a sudden development of oligohydramnios was noted. At 33 weeks' gestation, a normal male infant was delivered by cesarean section. Although placental dysfunction could explain the decrease in amniotic fluid secretion, such acute changes should have caused fetal distress which was not observed. Hence, these findings suggested that cisplatin crossed the placenta and may have caused a decrease in fetal renal function. Creatinine levels were not obtained until three weeks after birth, at which time they were in the normal range described for his gestational age. One of cisplatin's major dose-limiting toxicities is renal damage and clinical trials of cisplatin in cancer patients have shown a high incidence of acute renal failure[28–30], although these effects can be partially controlled with adequate hydration. Animal studies have also shown cisplatin-induced nephrotoxicity[31].

We have recently documented that protein binding of platinum in infants and pregnant women is lower than in nonpregnant controls[32]. There is significant correlation between serum albumin concentrations and cisplatin protein binding, with infants having lower levels and hence, higher concentrations of the free drug. It is therefore conceivable that pregnant women have higher level of free drug. It is the free fraction of drug that crosses the placenta. The higher levels of free drugs in the mother and fetus may increase the risk of nephrotoxicity in both.

Antimetabolites

Antimetabolites are synthetic drugs that act by interfering with the synthesis of DNA, RNA, and some important coenzymes (for example, dihydrofolate reductase). As structural analogs of precursor purine and pyrimidine bases, they are incorporated into DNA and ultimately lead to nonfunctional DNA and cell death. Antimetabolites act in the S phase (DNA synthesis phase) of the cell life cycle[9].

Aminopterin

Aminopterin, a folic acid antagonist, has been used as both abortifacient and chemotherapeutic agent[6]. It is no longer used as a chemotherapeutic agent.

Aminopterin induced central nervous system defects, cleft lip, and other skeletal defects in rats. In lambs, ear and skeletal defects have been reported and in primates abortion was induced[11].

In humans, aminopterin has been shown to increase the rate of fetal malformations. There are at least 16 documented cases of teratogenic effect of the drug when used alone[11]. The "aminopterin syndrome" of congenital anomalies is characterized by cranial depostosis (delay of ossification of the bones of the calvarium), hypertelorism wide nasal bridge, and anomalies of the external ears and micrognathia[33]. Schardein[11] reports that there have been a number of normal pregnancies following failure of abortion with aminopterin treatment; the estimated risk of malformation is about 1 : 3.

Methotrexate

Methotrexate is a folic acid antagonist that is closely related to aminopterin[33]. It has been found to be teratogenic in rats, mice, rabbits, and cats[1].

Schardein[1] reported on three pregnancies where there was first trimester exposure to methotrexate. In two cases, malformed skulls were reported and, in all three, there were abnormalities of the ears.

Methotrexate is also used in the treatment of rheumatoid arthritis[34]. In a study that looked at the first trimester exposure to low dose methotrexate in eight patients (ten pregnancies) with rheumatoid arthritis there were five full-term babies, three spontaneous abortions, and two therapeutic abortions. All offspring were of normal height and weight at birth with no physical abnormalities. The authors failed to demonstrate that methotrexate was teratogenic but the possibility of inducing spontaneous abortions remained. However, the dose of methotrexate used in collagen diseases is substantially lower than in cancer protocols, potentially explaining these differences. The risk of malformations from the drug was estimated at 1 : 4[1].

6-Mercaptopurine (6-MP)

6-mercaptopurine is a purine analog of hypoxanthine[8]. In the mouse, 6-MP is a chromosome breaker[11].

Sokan and Lessmann[5] report on three cases where 6-MP was used in the first trimester. In the first case, 6-MP was used from conception to seven months' gestation. The baby was born prematurely and died 19 hours after birth. The autopsy reported a normal premature infant. In the second case, 6-MP was used alternately with busulfan. The baby was born small with cleft palate, bilateral ocular defects, and hypoplasia of the thyroid and ovaries. She died two months after birth. In the third case, 6-MP was used until six months' gestation with aminopterin and desacetylmethylcolchicine beginning in the fourth and sixth month, respectively. The mother delivered spontaneously at six months gestation. The baby lived for only 19 hours but was born with no malformations.

Diamond *et al*[24] reported on a woman who received 400 rad to her spleen at one month gestation and 100 mg/day 6-MP throughout the entire pregnancy. She delivered a premature infant at 36 weeks' gestation who was alive and well.

In total, there are now over 100 cases of 6-MP exposure in humans during embryogenesis with no apparent increased teratogenic risk[1].

Cytosine arabinoside (ARA-C)

Cytosine arabinoside is an analog of the nucleoside deoxycytidine and is phosphorylated to Ara-cytosine triphosphate (Ara-CTP). Ara-CTP is a competitive inhibitor of DNA polymerase[8]. In rats, Ara-C causes cleft palate, tail, limb and digit defects, and fetal death[11,35].

Ara-C and thioguanine were administered as a maintenance program to a woman with leukemia throughout pregnancy. The pregnancy was uncomplicated and she delivered a male infant at 38 weeks' gestation with distal limb defects. The medial two digits of his feet were missing as well as the distal phalanges of both thumbs. This patient subsequently became pregnant again while being on the same dosages of Ara-C and thioguanine throughout this pregnancy. This time she delivered a term female infant whose physical findings were entirely normal[36]. This case illustrates the unpredictable effect of chemotherapy on the fetus early in pregnancy.

In another case, a leukemic woman was treated several times early in her pregnancy with the drug Ara-C. The male infant was born with limb deformities[11]. The estimated relative risk of malformations is 1:8[11].

5-Flurouracil (5-FU)

5-FU is a pyrimidine antagonist[37]. It has induced multiple malformations in mice, rats, rabbits, guinea pigs, and hamsters. In primates, 5-FU has caused rib and vertebral anomalies[11].

Barber[4] describes a woman with advanced breast cancer who received 5-FU for the first three months of pregnancy. She delivered a normal infant. In contrast, Stephens *et al*[37] reported on a woman with an intestinal malignancy who was treated at 11 weeks' gestation with intravenous 5-FU five times per week for one month. A therapeutic abortion was performed at 16 weeks. The fetus was affected by multiple congenital anomalies including absent thumbs and fingers, hypoplastic aorta, pulmonary hypoplasia, and an absent appendix. The estimated risk to malformation was 1:3[11].

Vinca alkaloids

Vinca alkaloids are agents that inhibit spindle formation by binding to tubulin and thus stop the cell from dividing[8]. They act mainly during the M phase.

Vincristine and vinblastine

Both vincristine and vinblastine have been shown to have an embryocidal effect in hamsters. Skeletal defects were also noted[38]. Hamster fetuses which were exposed to vincristine had malformations including microphthalmia, anophthalmia, mild exencephaly, and rib defects. Vinblastine produced malformations including microphthalmia, anophthalmia, spina bifida, and skeletal defects.

Vinblastine administration during the first trimester produced no malformations in ten infants as reported by Scharpia and Chudley[39]. In addition, a woman who was treated with vinblastine throughout her pregnancy also delivered a normal infant[40]. No congenital malformations were noted in babies of 11 women treated with vincristine during pregnancy; three of these women were treated in the first trimester[21].

Antibiotics

Doxorubicin inhibits DNA and DNA-dependent RNA synthesis by binding to DNA and untwisting the helix[8]. Doxorubicin produces malformations in rats, but not in mice or rabbits. This difference may be due to metabolic differences[11].

In humans, none of the chemotherapeutic antibiotic drugs have been associated with birth defects[1]. Doxorubicin, in combination with cyclophosphamide and 5-FU, was given to a woman at 11 weeks of pregnancy. She received six courses of this therapy and then the doxorubicin was replaced by methotrexate for the remainder of the pregnancy. She delivered a 35 weeks' gestation female infant with no evidence of any abnormality. Following-up at 24 months showed normal growth and development[41].

Combination chemotherapy

The apparent rate of fetal malformation associated with combination chemotherapy is similar to the rate observed with single agents (16% vs 17%, respectively). However, excluding folate antagonists and concurrent radiation therapy, the estimated incidence of fetal malformation with single agents drops to 6%[33].

It should be noted in all the above estimations of teratogenic risks that the figures are based on summaries of case reports and small series. This approach is fraught with the risk of reporting bias (which tends to over-report adverse effects) and poor description of fetal outcome.

Malformations in infants whose mothers received chemotherapy during the second and third trimesters occur very rarely at rates that are comparable to the general population[2,6].

Other toxic effects

The administration of cytotoxic drugs to women during the second or third trimester may result in abortion, stillbirth or growth retardation[33]. Of the newborns, 40% are estimated to have low birth weight[2].

The systemic toxicity of chemotherapy on the neonates is not known. Few reports associate this mode of treatment with hematopoietic depression, which is self-limiting, usually within weeks but nevertheless increases the risk of neonatal infection and hemorrhage[18,40–44]. In addition, hormonal alteration, such as adrenal insufficiency from prolonged corticosteroid therapy has also been reported[45].

Very little information is available on delayed effects of *in utero* exposure to antineoplastic agents. Long-term studies are needed to confirm or reject suggestions that children born to mothers who were treated by chemotherapy during pregnancy might have impaired mental and physical development and infertility[43,44,46,47]. To date, only one study measures long term developmental outcome specifically. Aviles and NIZ[48] examined 17 offspring of women treated for acute leukemia during pregnancy. Neurological, intellectual and visual–motor–perceptual assessments were administered to the offspring who ranged in age from 4 to 22 years as well as to their siblings and to unrelated controls. No differences in developmental scores were detected among the groups. Although interpretation of the findings are constrained by the lack of presentation of data, the question as to whether the children were assessed "blind" and the use of cross-sectional rather than longitudinal design, the study is important as the only existing examination of developmental outcome following exposure *in utero* to cytotoxic therapy.

In addition, studies should evaluate the incidence of second malignancies in these children. Chemotherapy, especially alkylating agents, is of proven carcinogenetic potential in adults[49]. For example, the risk of developing a second malignancy during or after therapy of ALL is high and estimated to be 62.3 per 100 000 annually[50]. Although the risk of exposure to chemotherapy *in utero* is theoretically high since most antineoplastic drugs cross the placenta, this may be counterbalanced by relatively few cycles of drugs that the mother usually receives during pregnancy[18]. Diethylstilbestrol treatment of pregnant women has been linked to late development of clear cell carcinoma of the vagina in young women[51]. The Toronto Leukemia Study Group reported that a son of a patient with ALL who was exposed *in utero* to cyclophosphamide and steroids, developed neuroblastoma arising from the adrenal gland at age 14 years and papillary carcinoma of the thyroid when he was 16 years old[41]. That his twin sister was not affected suggests pharmacogenetic predisposition to the effects of cyclophosphamide. No other cases of malignancies have been reported.

Summary

The occurrence of cancer during pregnancy is extremely stressful to both patient and physician. It poses a conflict between optimal diagnostic workup and treatment of the mother and the potential adverse effects they may have on fetal well-being. This issue is even more complicated since the number of reported cases of pregnancy and cancer is small and the current management strategies are based on anecdotal reports.

Animal studies reveal that almost all antineoplastic agents are teratogenic but extrapolation to human malformations is not simple because of species differences. Although cytotoxic drugs damage both DNA and RNA, their use in pregnant women poses small risk of congenital malformations to their offspring. This risk is especially evident in fetuses exposed to cytotoxic drugs during the first trimester and is estimated to be approximately 10%. Treatment of women during the subsequent trimesters has not been associated with increased risk fetal malformations.

To date, only aminopterin, which is not used anymore, had been definitely linked to a homogenous pattern of fetal malformations when used during the first trimester of pregnancy. However, although based mainly on sporadic case reports, other antimetabolites (methotrexate) should be omitted from drug regimen of pregnant women during the first trimester.

It should be pointed out that other toxic effects must be taken into consideration in the treatment of the pregnant women with chemotherapy. For example, hematopoietic suppression imposes higher risk of infection and bleeding to both the mother and the fetus. Long-term studies are needed to evaluate the effects of chemotherapy administered to mothers during pregnancy on children's mental and physical development, infertility and the occurrence of second malignancies.

References

1. Schardein JL: Cancer chemotherapeutic agents. In *Chemically Induced Birth Defects*, (Schardein JL, ed.) 2nd ed. 1993; pp. 457–508, 1993, Marcel Dekker Inc., New York.
2. Nicholson HO: Cytotoxic drugs in pregnancy: review of reported cases. *J Obstet Gynecol Br Comonw* 1968; 75: 307–12.
3. Kalter H, Warkany J: Congenital malformations. *N Engl J Med* 1983; 308: 424–31, 491–7.
4. Barber HRK: Fetal and neonatal effects of cytotoxic agents. *Obstet Gynecol* 1981; 58: 41S–7S.
5. Sokal JE, Lessmann EM: Effects of cancer chemotherapeutic agents on the human fetus. *JAMA* 1960; 172(16): 1765–72.
6. Sutcliffe SB: Treatment of neoplastic disease during pregnancy: maternal and fetal effects. *Clin Invest Med* 1985; 8: 333–8.
7. Gallenberg MM, Loprinzi CL: Breast cancer and pregnancy. *Semin Oncol* 1989; 16(5): 369–6.
8. Erlichman C, Kerr IG: Antineoplastic drugs. In *Principles of Medical Pharmacology* (Kalant H, Roschlau WHE, eds.) 1989; pp. 604–614, BC Decker Inc., Toronto.
9. Krepart GV, Lotocki RJ: Chemotherapy during pregnancy. In *Cancer in Pregnancy* (Allen HH, Nisker JA, ed.) 1985; pp. 69–88, Futura Publishing Co. Inc. Mt Kisco New York.
10. Garrett MJ: Teratogenic effects of combination chemotherapy. *Ann Int Med* 1974; 80: 667.
11. Schardein JL: Cancer chemotherapeutic agents. In *Chemically Induced Birth Defects*. (Schardein JL, ed.) 1985, pp. 467–520, Marcel Dekker Inc. New York.
12. Moore MJ: Clinical pharmacokinetics of cyclophosphamide. *Clin Pharmacokinet* 1991; 20(3): 194–208.
13. Hales BF: Comparison of the mutagenicity and teratogenicity of cyclophosphamide and its active metabolites, 4-hydrocyclophosphamide, phosphoramide mustard, and acrolein. *Cancer Res* 1982; 42: 3016–21.
14. Mirkes PE, Fantel AG, Reenaway JC, Shepeard TH: Teratogenicity of cyclophosphamide metabolites: phosphoramide mustard, acrolein, and 4-ketocyclophosphamide in rat embryos cultured *in vitro*. *Toxical Apple Pharmacol* 1981; 58: 322–30.
15. Speilmann H, Jacob-Muller V: Investigations on cyclophosphamide treatment during the pre-implantation period. II. *In vitro* studies on the effects of cyclophosphamide and its metabolites 4-OH-cyclophosphamide, phosphoramide mustard, and acroline on blastulation of 4-cell and 8-cell mouse embryos and on their subsequent development during implantation. *Teratology*, 1981; 23: 7–13.
16. Greenberg LH, Tanaka KR: Congenital anomalies probably induced by cyclophosphamide. *JAMA* 1964; 188(5): 123–6.

17. Toledo TM, Harper RC, Moser RH: Fetal effects during cyclophosphamide and irradiation therapy. *Ann Int Med* 1971; 74: 87–91.
18. Reynoso EE, Shepherd FA, Messner HA, Farquharson HA, Garvey MB, Baker MA: Acute leukemia during pregnancy: the Toronto Leukemia study group experience with long-term follow-up of children exposed *in utero* to chemotherapeutic agents. *J Clin Oncol* 1987; 5(7): 1098–106.
19. Zemlickis DM, Lishner M, Erlich R, Koren G: Teratogenicity and carcinogenicity in a twin exposed *in utero* to cyclophosphamide. *Teratogenesis, Carcinogen Mutagen* 1993; 13: 139–43.
20. Shetton D, Monie IW: Possible teratogenic effect of chlorambucil on a human fetus. *JAMA* 1963; 186(1): 180–1.
21. Gililland J, Weinstein L: The effects of cancer chemotherapeutic agents on the developing fetus. *Obstet Gynecol Surv* 1983; 38: 6–13.
22. Dugdale M, Fort AT: Busulfan treatment of leukemia during pregnancy. *JAMA* 1967; 199(2): 167–9.
23. Dennis LH, Stein S: Busulfan in pregnancy. *JAMA* 1965; 192(9): 131–2.
24. Diamond I, Anderson MM, McCreadie SR: Transplacental transmission of busulfan (Myeran®) in a mother with leukemia. *Pediatrics* 1960; 25: 85–90.
25. Abramovici A, Shaklai M, Pinkhas J: Myeloschisis in a six weeks embryo of a leukemia woman treated by busulfan. *Teratology* 1978; 18: 241–6.
26. Beaudoin AR, Connely TG: Teratogenic studies with platinum thymine blue. *Teratology* 1978; 17: 46A–7A.
27. Jacobs AJ, Marchevsky A, Gordon RE, Deppe G, Cohen CJ: Oat cell carcinoma of the uterine cervix in a pregnant woman; treatment with cicdiamminedichloroplatinum. *Gynecol Oncol* 1980; 9: 405–10.
28. Weiner MW, Jacobs C: Mechanism of cisplatin nephrotoxicity. *FASEB* 1983; 42: 2974–8.
29. Fillastre JP, Raguenez-Viotle G: Cisplatin nephrotoxicity. *Toxicol Lett* 1989; 46: 163–75.
30. Reis F, Klastersky J: Nephrotoxicity induced by cancer chemotherapy with special emphasis on cisplatin toxicity. *Am J Kid Dis* 1986; 8: 368–79.
31. Kociba RJ, Sleight SD: Acute toxicologic and pathologic effects of cisdiamminedichloroplatinum (NSC-119875) in the male rat. *Cancer Chemother Repiatr* 1971; 55: 1–9.
32. Zemlickis D, Klein J, Moselhy G, Koren G: Cisplatin protein binding in pregnancy and the neonatal period. *Pediatr Med Oncol* 1994;
33. Doll DC, Ringenberg QS, Yarbro JW: Antineoplastic agents and pregnancy. *Semin Oncol* 1989; 16(5): 337–46.
34. Kozlowski RD, Steinbrunner JV, MacKenzie AH, Clough JD, Wilke WS, Segal AM: Outcome of first-trimester exposure to low-dose methotrexate in eight pateints with rheumatic disease. *Am J Med* 1990; 88: 589ø2.
35. Pawlinger DF, McLean FW, Noyes WD: Normal fetus after cytosine arabinoside therapy. *Ann Intern Med* 1971; 74(6): 1012.
36. Schafer AI: Teratogenic effects of antileukemic chemotherapy. *Arch Intern Med* 1981; 141: 514–15.
37. Stephens JD, Golbus MS, Miller TR, Wilber RR, Epstein CJ: Multiple congenital anomalies in a fetus exposed to 5-flurouracil during the first trimester. *Am J Obstet Gynecol* 1980; 137: 746–9.
38. Ferm VH: Congenital malformations in hamster embryos after treatment with vinblastine and vicristine. *Science* 1963; 141: 426.
39. Schapira DV, Chudley AE: Successful pregnancy following continuous

treatment with combination chemotherapy before conception and throughout pregnancy. *Cancer* 1984; 54: 800–3.

40. Armstrong JG, Dyke RW, Fouts PH: Vinblastine sulphate treatment of Hodgkin's diseases during pregnancy. *Science* 1964; 143: 703.

41. Turchi JJ, Villasis C: Antihacyclines in the treatment of malignancy in pregnancy. *Cancer* 1988; 61: 435–40.

42. Finkbeiner JA: Antineoplastic chemotherapy in pregnancy. In *Surgical Disease in Pregnancy.* (Barber HKK, Graber EA, eds.), 1974, pp. 711, WB Saunders Co., Philadelphia.

43. Sweet DL Jr., Kinzie J: Consequences of radiotherapy and anti-neoplastic therapy for the fetus. *J Reprod Med* 1976; 17: 241–6.

44. Blatt J, Mulvihill JJ, Ziegler JL *et al*: Pregnancy outcome following cancer chemotherapy. *Am J Med* 1980; 69: 828–32.

45. Globus MS: Teratology for the obstetrician: current status. *Obstet Gynecol* 1980; 55: 269–77.

46. Williams SF, Bitran JD: Cancer and pregnancy. *Clin Perinatol* 1985; 12: 609–23.

47. Andrien JM, Ochoa Molina E: Menstrual cycle, pregnancies and offspring before and after MOPP therapy for Hodgkin's disease. *Cancer* 1983; 52: 435–8.

48. Aviles A, Niz J: Long term followup of children born to mothers with acute leukemia in pregnancy. 1988; 16: 3–6.

49. Kyle RA: Second malignancies associated with chemotherapy. In *Toxicity of Chemotherapy* (Perry MC, Yarbo JW, ed.), 1984, pp. 479–506, Grune & Stratton, New York.

50. Ochs J, Mulhern RK: Late effects of antileukemic treatment. *Pediatr Clin N Am* 1988; 35: 815–33.

51. Herbst AL, Ulfeldert H, Poskanzer DC: Adenocarcinoma of the vagina. Association of maternal stilbestrol therapy with tumor appearance in young women. *N Engl J Med* 1971; 284: 878–81.

18

Fetal outcome following *in utero* exposure to cancer chemotherapy: the Toronto Study

D ZEMLICKIS, M. LISHNER, P. DEGENDORFER,
T. PANZARELLA, S. B. SUTCLIFFE AND
G. KOREN

Cancer is the second leading cause of death among women during the reproductive years[1,2]. Its occurrence during pregnancy is rare with an incidence of 0.07% to 0.1%[3,4]. Over the years, significant advances have been made with current chemotherapeutic agents in increasing longevity and improving survival. Cures and long-term remissions are obtained in diseases that previously were untreatable[5]. Oncologists, therefore, may be posed with a difficult challenge when a patient requires chemotherapy during pregnancy or becomes pregnant during the course of chemotherapy.

Although there are a variety of studies on the effects of chemotherapy during pregnancy on the fetus, review of the literature reveals that most reports are based on single cases[1,6,7], cohorts with small sample sizes[8] and cohorts that supply incomplete evaluation of the offspring[9].

Due to the rarity of chemotherapy use in pregnancy, it is unlikely that prospective studies will be undertaken. We therefore performed an historical cohort study to evaluate the effects of chemotherapy during pregnancy on fetal outcome, among women treated in the Princess Margaret Hospital (PMH) in Toronto between 1958 and 1947. We hypothesized that babies exposed to chemotherapeutic agents during the first trimester, when organogenesis takes place, may be more likely to suffer from major malformations than babies not exposed to chemotherapy or those exposed at subsequent trimesters. In addition, we hypothesized that suboptimal conditions in women with cancer receiving chemotherapy may increase the risk for spontaneous abortions, stillbirth, and lower birthweight for gestational age.

Methods

Cases with cancer in pregnancy who received chemotherapy while pregnant were extracted from the Princess Margaret Hospital's data base. For the purposes of this chapter, chemotherapy is considered also to include corticosteroids, hormone therapy, and biological response modifiers.

Details of the cancer, cancer staging, and date of diagnosis were recorded for the cases. All cases were rated by various staging systems as defined by the TNM system of 1987[10]. Charts with an ambiguous staging were assessed from their pathology reports and clinical workup.

Dates and types of treatment were obtained. For obstetrical information, date of conception, gestational age at diagnosis and first treatment, complications in pregnancy, if any, and pregnancy outcome were recorded.

For pregnancies that continued to term or resulted in stillbirth, birth records were requested from the delivering hospital. For live births, sex and birthweight of the infant were recorded, as well as gestational age at delivery, type of delivery, Apgar scores, fetal complications, and congenital anomalies. In the case of a cesarean section, the reason for choosing this method was recorded. For intrauterine death, date of diagnosis of the still-birth and autopsy results were collected.

Fetal outcome after *in utero* exposure to chemotherapy was compared to that of babies born to women attending the Motherisk clinic during the first trimester following exposure to drugs, chemicals, or radiation during pregnancy[11]. For this analysis, each mother who received chemotherapy and had a live birth was matched to a mother of similar age who was not exposed to teratogenic drugs or chemicals[12,13].

To detect whether any differences in mean birth weight between cases and the Motherisk control group were due to differences in gestational age or small birth weight, birth weights were plotted on a standardized percentile curve according to gestational age[14].

Results

There were 21 cases of women treated with chemotherapy during pregnancy identified in the 30 years analyzed in our study. The mean age of cancer treated pregnant women was 27.4 $\pm$ 6.6 years at diagnosis, with a median age of 28.5 years (range 14 to 41).

Of the 21 pregnancies, 5 women had breast cancer, 4 Hodgkin's disease, 4 melonoma, 4 leukemia (2 AML and 2 CML), 2 non-Hodgkin's lymphoma, 1 ovarian, and 1 case of rhabdomyosarcoma.

Types of chemotherapy, gestational age at time of exposure, and outcome of the pregnancy are presented in Table 18.1. Of those women who were exposed to chemotherapy during the first trimester ($n = 13$), five women maintained the pregnancy to term, four had a spontaneous

Table 18.1. *Pregnancy outcome following administration of chemotherapeutic agents during pregnancy*

Case	Maternal diagnosis	Agents	Results and comments
First trimester exposure			
1	Breast	1,2,3	S.A.
2	Breast	4	S.A.
3	Breast	1,2,3,5,6	Live birth aaw
4	HD	7	S.A.
5	HD	7	T.A.
6	HD	7	Hydrocephaly, died 4 h after birth
7	Mel	8	T.A.
8	Mel	9	T.A.
9	Mel	10	Live birth aaw
10	Mel	8	Blue baby at birth, died at 8 months
11	NHL	11	S.A.
12	CML	12,13,14,15	T.A.
13	CML	16	Live birth aaw
14	NHL	1,5,20	T.A.
15	AML	17,14,15	Still birth at 26 weeks. Born with bruising and petechiae over multiple areas
17	Rhabdo	18	Addicted to Brompton's cocktail Live birth SGA, normal otherwise
18	Breast	3,17,1,6	Live birth aaw
19	Breast	1,2,3	Live birth aaw, SGA
20	HD	20	Live birth aaw
21	Ovary	1,17,19	Live birth aaw

[a]1 = cyclophosphamide, 2 = methotrexate, 3 = 5FU, 4 = melphalon, 5 = vincristine, 6 = tamoxifen, 7 = MOPP (nitrogen mustard, vincristine, predisone, procarbazine), 8 = BCG (Bacillus Calmette–Guerin), 9 = DTIC (dimethyl triazeno imidazole carboxamide), 10 = levamisole, 11 = 6-mercaptopurine, 12 = daunomycin, 13 = hydroxyurea, 14 = cytosine arabinoside, 15 = 6-thioguanine, 16 = Myleran, 17 = Adriamycin, 18 = essiac, 19 = *cis*-platinum, 20 = prednisone
Note: HD = Hodgkin's disease, Mel = melanoma, NHL = non-Hodgkin's lymphoma, CML = chronic mylogenous leukemia, AML = acute mylogenous leukemia, Rhabdo = rhabdomyosarcoma, S.A. = spontaneous abortion, aaw = alive and well, TA = therapeutic abortion, SGA = small for gestational age.

abortion, and four had a therapeutic abortion. Two of those pregnancies exposed to chemotherapy resulted in major malformation. In one case, the child died of hydrocephaly after birth; the mother used MOPP four weeks into the pregnancy for stage 4B Hodgkin's disease. The postmortem report did not disclose the definitive pathology leading to the hydrocephalus. The other baby had severe cardiac problems with a patent ductus arteriosus and a ventricular septal defect. The pulmonary valve was either defective or absent. The baby died at 8 months following cardiac surgery. The mother had been exposed to Bacille Calmette–Guerin (BCG) until 4 weeks into the gestation for stage 1 Clarke's level 3 melanoma.

Four women had chemotherapy during the second trimester, resulting in two live births, one stillbirth, and one therapeutic abortion. One baby, born to a mother with rhabdomyosarcoma, was small at birth, addicted to Brompton's cocktail, but was normal otherwise. Brompton's cocktail is a mixture of cocaine and morphine sulfate suspended in chloroform or tap water. The mother also had been receiving Essiac, an experimental drug, at 20 weeks of gestation at another institution. Essiac is an aqueous infusion of four botanical herbs: *Arctium lappa* (burdock), *Ulmus fulva* (slippery elm), *Rheum palmatum* (Indian rhubarb) and *Rumex actosa* (sorrell). Essiac has not been considered as an investigational drug and has not been approved for study in further clinical trials[15].

Of interest is the case of stillbirth of the mother who was diagnosed with acute myologenous leukemia at 23 weeks of gestation. At the time of diagnosis, the oncologist noted that there was good fetal movement and a fetal heart beat was heard. The mother was treated for 7 days with adriamycin, cytosine arabinoside, and 6-thioguanine starting at 24 weeks' gestation. Nine days after the end of the chemotherapy, she had a stillbirth which appeared to be normal on examination with the exception of multiple areas of brusing and petechiae.

All four pregnancies exposed to chemotherapy during the third trimester resulted in a live birth with no complications or malformations.

Of the 21 pregnancies studied, there were 12 deliveries (1 was a stillbirth), 5 therapeutic abortions, and 4 spontaneous abortions. We were able to obtain ten obstetrical records from the delivering hospitals. One obstetrical report and the autopsy report could not be obtained because the delivering hospitals had destroyed the birth records. A summary of the available information regarding fetal outcome is presented in Table 18.2.

There was a statistically lower mean birth weight for babies of mothers who received chemotherapy during pregnancy when compared to their matched controls (p < 0.001). Similarly, they had a statistically shorter mean gestation age (p = 0.0056) due to a significantly higher proportion of preterm deliveries, mainly due to induced labor to allow more aggressive maternal treatment.

To assess whether the lower birth weight in babies of cancer patients was due to a greater proportion of premature births or due to smaller birth weight, the distribution of birth weight percentiles (corrected for gestational

Table 18.2. *Comparison of fetal outcome in mothers who received chemotherapy during pregnancy to the matched control group[c]*

	n	Study babies	*n*	Matched control babies
Mean gestaional age	11	36.4 ± 4.2 weeks[a]	11	40.8 ± 1.3 weeks[a]
Number of preterm births (< 37 weeks)	11	5	11	0
Mean birth weight	9	2227 ± 558 g[b]	11	3519 ± 272 g[b]
Delivery method	11	6 spontaneous 5 cesarean	11	10 spontaneous 1 cesarean

[a]p $= 0.0056$.
[b]p $= \; < 0.001$.
[c]Plus–minus values are means $\pm$ SD.

age) was compared between the study and control groups. This analysis shows that babies born to women who received chemotherapy during pregnancy were significantly more likely to be below the 50th percentile (p < 0.01) (Table 18.3).

Discussion

The diagnosis of cancer during pregnancy poses a difficult challenge to the woman, her family, and the physicians caring for her because therapy of her cancer may be detrimental to the unborn baby. Equally important, a delay in diagnosis or treatment may compromise maternal survival. The mother may find it necessary to therapeutically terminate pregnancy or risk miscarriage or fetal damage because of chemotherapeutic treatment. These decisions may be very difficult because chemotherapy may diminish reproductive function[17]. These decisions may be easier if based on large experience; however, as the incidence of cancer occurring during pregnancy is rare (0.77% to 0.1%), large prospective studies are impractical[3,4].

To date, most studies on fetal outcome following chemotherapy, have methodological problems which make them difficult to interpret. A small sample size[8], single case reports[1,18], and incomplete records of fetal outcome are common[19,20]. The present study is the first to obtain fetal information and to compare it to matched control babies. However, although this study examines a complete cohort encompassing 26 years, the numbers are still quite small, with a heterogeneous group of diseases and treatments.

Most chemotherapeutic agents have been shown to inflict damage to

Table 18.3. *Distribution of birth weight percentiles in the study and control groups*

	n	< 25th %ile	25th–50th %ile	50–75th %ile	75th–90th %ile	> 90th %ile
		Birth weight percentile for gestational age at delivery				
Cases[a]	9	5	2	1	1	0
Matched controls[a]	11	0	2	5	4	0

[a]p < 0.01.

rapidly dividing cells such as bone marrow, intestinal epithelium, and the reproductive organs[21]. Animal studies suggest that, similarly, the fetus would be sensitive to these agents as fetal tissues have a high growth rate. This may result in spontaneous abortions or malformations[21].

Garrett reported on a child delivered at 24 weeks with abnormalities of both feet, the right tibia, and a cerebral hemorrhage[7]. The mother had received nitrogen mustard, vinblastine, prednisone, and procarbazine during the first trimester. In our study, a child whose mother was exposed to nitrogen mustard, vincristine, prednisone, and provcarbazine, died of hydrocephaly after birth.

As the use of BCG is not common in the prevention of tuberculosis, there is little information on its use in pregnancy[22]. One baby in our study died of cardiac malformations after being exposed to BCG during the first trimester. It is not possible to establish the causation of these malformations. However, unlike chemotherapy, the ability of BCG to destroy growing cells is not biologically plausible.

While exposure to chemotherapy in the first trimester has been associated with major malformations of the fetus, exposure during the second and third trimesters does not result in structural malformations[3,8,21], but may affect birth weight[23] or the CNS which develops throughout pregnancy. Long-term developmental effects of chemotherapy are not addressed in the present study, and would be valuable extension of our analysis. Our study did not detect major malformations in children of women exposed to cancer chemotherapy during the second and third trimesters. Conversely, one woman exposed to cytosine arabinoside, 6-thioguanine, and adriamycin during the second trimester had a stillbirth; the baby had petechiae and brusing which may reflect severe thrombocytopenia secondary to bone marrow suppression; conversely, these findings are commonly seen in preterm babies born at 26 weeks of gestation. Our cohort of babies exposed to chemotherapy during the first trimester and continued to term is too small to prove increased teratogenic risk; yet, only in this group were there major malformations, whereas babies exposed to chemotherapy later in gestation were all morphologically normal.

Analysis of outcome of all 223 cases of cancer in pregnancy shows a significantly higher risk of stillbirth. Because the vast majority of these women did not receive chemotherapy, it is probable that maternal cancer caused suboptimal intrauterine conditions and increased risk of stillbirth. This hypothesis is supported by our observation of significantly low birthweight for gestational age associated with chemotherapy during pregnancy. It is conceivable that women who needed chemotherapy in pregnancy represent a subgroup with more severe degrees of cancer. Similar results were found by us in a study in which low birth weight for gestational age was associated with breast cancer during pregnancy[24]. The association between low birth weight for gestational age and stillbirth has long been recognized[13].

Intrauterine growth restriction (IUGR) is defined as either asymmetric growth using a ponderal index or by weight less than 10th percentile for gestational age. In our cohort there was a tendency to deliver the babies at an earlier gestational age, to allow more aggressive maternal treatment. However, even after correction for gestational age, the babies exposed *in utero* to chemotherapy were of significantly lower percentile for their age. Although only few of them satisfy the definition of IUGR, the systematic tendency for lower birth weights reflects suboptimal intrauterine growth.

In summary, our study confirms the increased likelihood of spontaneous abortions and major birth defects when chemotherapy is used during embryogenesis, whereas such a risk is not apparent beyond the first trimester. The case of stillbirth is consistent with direct toxic effects of multiple drug therapy on the fetus. Because of the higher risk for stillbirth and low birth weight for gestational age, women with cancer should be followed closely by a high risk obstetrical unit, to define the optimal time of delivery.

References

1. Gililland J, Weinstein L: The effects of cancer chemotherapeutic agents on the developing fetus. *Obstet Gynecol Surv.* 1983; 38: 6–13.
2. Silverberg E, Lubera J: Cancer statistics 1986. *CA* 1986; 36: 9–25.
3. Sutcliffe SB: Treatment of neoplastic diseases during pregnancy: maternal and fetal effects. *Clin Invest Med* 1985; 8: 333–8.

 4. Potter JF, Schoeneman M: Metastasis of maternal cancer to the placenta and fetus. *Cancer* 1970; 25: 380–8.
 5. DeVita VT Jr: The consequences of the chemotherapy of Hodgkin's disease. *Cancer* 1981; 47: 1–13.
 6. Schapira DV, Chudley AE: Successful pregnancy following continuous treatment with combination chemotherapy before conception and throughout pregnancy. *Cancer* 1984; 54: 800–3.
 7. Garrett MJ: Teratogenic effects of combination chemotherapy (Letter). *Ann Intern Med* 1974; 80(5): 667.
 8. Blatt J, Mulvihill JJ, Ziegler JL, Young RC, Poplack DG: Pregnancy outcome following cancer chemotherapy. *Am J Med* 1980; 69: 828–32.
 9. Mulvihill JJ, McKeen EA, Rosner F, Zarrabi MH: Pregnancy outcome in cancer patients. *Cancer* 1987; 60: 1143–50.
10. Hermanek P, Sobin LH (eds.): *TNM Classification of Malignant Tumors*, 4th ed. 1987, Springer-Verlag, New York.
11. Koren G, MacLeod SM: Monitoring and avoiding drug and chemical teratogenicity. *Can Med Assoc J* 1986; 135: 1079–81.
12. Koren G: *Maternal–Fetal Toxicology: A Clinician's Guide* 1990, pp. 15–27, Marcel-Dekker, New York.
13. Schlesslman JJ: Basic methods of analysis. In *Case-Control Studies: Design, Conduct, Analysis* (Lilienfled AM, ed.) pp. 171–226, 1982, Oxford University Press, New York.
14. Brenner WE, Edelmand DA, Hendricks CH: A standard of fetal growth for the United States of America. *Am J Obstet Gynecol* 1976; 126: 555–64.
15. Yamamoto, A: Essiac. *Can J Hosp Pharm* 1988; 41(3): 158.
16. Registrar General of Ontario: Province of Ontario Vital Statistics: Table E, 'Summary of Live Births, Live Births to Unmarried Mothers and Stillbirths, and Rates, Ontario.' vols 1960 to 1985.
17. Gradishar WJ, Schilsky RL: Ovarian function following radiation and chemotherapy for cancer. *Semin Oncol* 1989; 16(5): 425–36.
18. O'Donnell R, Costigan C, O'Connell LG: Two cases of acute leukaemia in pregnancy. *Acta Haemat* 1979; 61: 298–300.
19. Nicholson HO: Cytotoxic drugs in pregnancy. Review of reported cases. *J Obstet Gynecol Br Commonw* 1968; 75: 307–12.
20. Sutton R, Buzdar AU, Hortobgyi GN: Pregnancy and offspring after adjuvant chemotherapy in breast cancer patients. *Cancer* 1990; 65(4): 847–50.
21. Sokal J, Lessmann EM: Effects of cancer chemotherapeutic agents on the human fetus. *JAMA* 1960; 172(16): 1765–72.
22. Amstey, MS: Vaccination in pregnancy. *Clin Obstet Gynecol* 1983; 10(1): 13–22.
23. Doll DC, Ringenberg QS, Yarbo JW: Management of cancer during pregnancy. *Arch Intern Med* 1988; 148: 2058–64.
24. Zemlickis D, Lishner M, Degendorfer P, Panzarella T, Burke B, Sutcliffe SB, Koren G: *Maternal and Fetal Outcome Following Breast Cancer in Pregnancy. Am J Obstet Gynecol* 1992; 166: 781–7.

19

Intrauterine causes of tumors in later life

G. KOREN

Today, there is a large body of evidence on *in utero* carcinogenesis in animal models (Table 19.1). However, the mechanisms underlying these processes are poorly understood. It is possible that the time window of carcinogenesis is dependent on activation of some compounds into active metabolites by either placenta (see Chapter 4) or target cells in the fetus. For a complete reference on existing experimental studies the reader may wish to refer to Schuller's recent book[1].

In this chapter we will focus on evidence existing today of transplacental human carcinogenicity, including proven as well as yet to be proven agents.

Diethylstilbestrol (DES)

In 1971, Herbst and colleagues published the first series of adenocarcinoma of the vagina in adolescent females exposed to the hormone during the first 10 weeks of fetal life[2]. The adenosis, cervical erosions and ridges were believed at that time to occur at very high frequency of exposed fetuses. However, as shown subsequently by the registry of DES cases, the risk of this cancer was less than one in thousands[3]! The causation was probably detected owing the extreme rarity of this tumor among adolescent girls.

On the other hand, morphological changes in the vaginal epithel could be detected in as many as 34% of exposed girls (compared to 0.4% in the general population). As shown in Table 18.1, similar changes could be reproduced in animal models. With the removal of DES from the market and the disappearance of this syndrome, it still remains an important milestone in understanding the molecular and cellular mechanisms leading to late carcinogenesis.

In males exposed to DES, no carcinogenesis has been demonstrated;

Table 19.1. *Examples of intrauterine carcinogenicity shown in animals.*

Compounds	Species	Tissues affected
Nitrosamides	Rats Hamsters	Brain, spina cord, nerves, endocrine system, digestive tract
Polycyclic aromatic hydrocarbone	Rats	Reticulosarcomas, malignant lipomas, lung, liver, marmana, kidney and brain tumors
	Hamsters	Skin, kidney, ovarian, thyroid and CNS tumors
Dialkylnitrosamines	Rats	Nephroblastoma, neuroepitheliomas, forestomach carcinoma, malignant neurinomas
Urethane	Hamsters	Malignant melanomas
DES	Hamsters	Metoplasia and neoplasia of male and female genital tract

however, abnormalities of the epididymis, cryptorchidism, hypogonadism and diminished spermatogenesis have been demonstrated.

Intrauterine exposure to phenytoin and the occurrence of neuroblastoma

During the last two decades, five cases of neuroblastoma have been reported in infants and young children exposed *in utero* to the antiepileptic drug phenytoin[4–9] (Table 19.2). After describing the fourth case in 1981, Ehrenbard and Chaganti stated that "it should take about 45 years for 4 cases of fetal hydantoin syndrome (FHS) with neuroblastoma to occur by chance; in fact it took no more than 5 years[8]." However, no more cases have been reported in the subsequent 7 years.

Recently, after diagnosing a case of neuroblastoma in an infant exposed to phenytoin *in utero* (see Case Report), we examined the potential association between intrauterine exposure to phenytoin and neuroblastoma using two research approaches: an *in vitro* lymphocyte toxicity assay for phenytoin-induced reactions and a case series of infants and children with neuroblastoma diagnosed over 17 years at our center.

Case report

An 18 year-old unmarried Caucasian woman (45 kg) suffering from grand mal epilepsy has been treated with phenytoin (Dilantin®) 200 mg twice

Table 19.2. *Reported cases of neuroblastoma in children exposed* in utero *to phenytoin*

Reference	Maternal age	Length of DPH[b] (yr)	Birth weight (kg)	Sex	Race	Postnatal problems	Age of Dx of neoplasm	Presenting symptoms
4	24	Since 10	2.950	F	n/a	Growth retardation	3 yr	Large abdominal tumor, below 3rd centile of weight and height, metopic suture ridging, hypertelorism, ptosis, epicanthal folds, fingerlike thumbs, hypoplasia of distal phalanges and nails.
5	n/a	Since 8	n/a	M	n/a	Growth retardation	7 d	Abdominal mass, hypertelorism, metopic ridging, malformed pinnae, single palmar creases, a third-degree hypospadias, mental retardation (parents retarded), reduced distal phalanges
6	27	1 yr	1.560	n/a	n/a	Gross mental and motor retardation	35 mo	35 mo hyperactivity, gross motor and mental retardation, hypertelorism, bilateral ptosis, increased epicanthal folds, high arched palate, frontal bossing, VSD[a]
7	30	25 yr	3.200	M	n/a	Progressive respiratory distress	1 d	Microcephaly, depressed nasal bridge, mild hypertelorism, normal shape and placement of ears, intact palate, transverse palmar creases, hypoplastic toe nails, small penis, VSD
8	25	7 yr	50 centile	M	n/a	n/a	35 mo	Mild motor and developmental delays, hypertelorism, microcephaly, epicanthal folds, small ears

[a]VSD, ventricular septal defect.
[b]DPH, diphenyl hydantoin.

daily (8.89 m/kg/day) since diagnosis at the age of 13 years. Her last seizure occurred after her first pregnancy (at age 17). The more recent conception occurred after discontinuing her oral contraceptive, and she continued the same dose of phenytoin throughout pregnancy. The 21 year-old father and mother are cigarette smokers (one package/day), and her father drinks alcohol heavily on weekends.

After an uneventful full-term pregnancy (40 weeks) with a weight gain of 11 kg, she gave birth vaginally to an apparently healthy female infant of 3.5 kg and head circumference of 36 cm. At 2 months of age, her measurements were weight, 4.9 kg; head circumference, 40 cm, and chest circumference, 37 cm. Poor feeding, difficulty in breathing, and abdominal fullness were noted at 4 weeks of age. Abdominal ultrasound revealed a left abdominal mass consistent with neuroblastoma, and at operation, a large neuroblastoma was resected.

An examination by a clinical geneticist was done at 6 months of age. Her height was 68 cm (90th centile); weight, 7.2 kg (25th centile); and head circumference, 43 cm (50th centile). She had no major malformations. Of note was some mild metopic ridging, brachycephaly, a glabellar capillary hemangioma, and a strawberry hemangioma on the left eyelid. Developmentally, she was age appropriate. Her distal digits were normal, and nails were hyperconvex but not hypoplastic. The dermatoglyphics were normal except for a distal axial triradius bilaterally.

The proband's half-brother (by a different father) was independently referred to the Genetics Clinic for assessment at 22 months of age. He was born at 41 weeks of gestation after an uneventful pregnancy with a birth weight of 3.3 kg. He was noted to have a left ptosis, which subsequently resolved. His general health had been good except for perennial rhinitis and a chronic eczematous skin condition responsive to topical corticosteroids. At age 19 months, he had an adenoidectomy, bilateral myringotomy, and tube placement. He had a developmental assessment at a chronological age of 20 months. His performance ranged from 16 to 22 months, and there was some concern about his speech development.

On examination at 22 months of age, his height and weight were between the 10th and 25th centiles. His head circumferences was 48 cm (50th centile). He had coarse hair, long thick eyelashes, a long philtrum, and overlapping helices of both ears. Both lobules were present.

He had a broad nasal bridge and maxillary hypoplasia but no cleft lip and palate. His alveolar ridges were broad, his neck short but was not webbed, and the hairline was normal. The cardiovascular examination was normal. Of note were the marked hypoplasia of the distal phalanges and triangular hypoplastic nails on the hands and feet. The dermatoglyphics were unusual and consistent with the hypoplastic digits. There were eight digital arches with the two remaining patterns being a small ulnar loop on each thumb. The resulting total distal ridge count was 8. There was distal axial triradium on the right palm and small whorl patterns on the plantar–hallucal areas.

In vitro *lymphocyte toxicity assay*

Lymphocytes of the patient, her half-brother, and mother were tested by an *in vitro* assay for phenytoin–metabolite-induced toxicity, which has been previously reported in detail[10,11]. Lymphocytes were prepared from whole blood with Ficoll–Paque and then suspended in a HEPES-buffered medium to yield 10^6 cells per reaction. Hepatic microsomes were prepared from National Institutes of Health General Purpose Swiss Mice [N:GP(SW)] pretreated with phenobarbital (10 mg/kg/body weight, given intraperitoneally for 3 days). Microsomal protein (0.28 mg) was incubated with the lymphocytes at 37 °C for 2 h along with 0.6 mM NADP, 2.4 mM glucose-6-phosphate, 2U of glucose-6-phosphate dehydrogenase, and phenytoin. A single concentration (62.5 μM) was chosen, which approximated *in vivo* conditions and which was derived from dose-toxicity studies. The drug was added in dimethyl sulfoxide (final concentrations, 2.5%). The same concentration of dimethyl sulfoxide was included in base-line samples lacking the drug. Cells were collected by centrifugation and resuspended in HEPES-buffered medium containing 5 mg of albumin per milliliter. Incubations were continued at 37 °C for 16 h, and aliquots then taken for lymphocyte viability assessment by trypan-blue dye exclusion. At least 200 cells were examined per sample in a blind protocol. Toxicity was reported as the difference in percent dead cells seen in the presence and absence of drug.

The response of the patient's lymphocytes (3% above baseline) was within the 99% confidence limits for normal phenytoin–metabolite lymphocyte response in control subjects. The response of lymphocytes of her epileptic mother and half-brother with FHS (5.4 and 6.2% above baseline, respectively) were in the intermediate range.

Case series

We reviewed the medical records at the Hospital for Sick Children in Toronto for cases diagnosed as neuroblastoma between January 1969 and October 1986. This hospital is the tertiary care center for all cases of neuroblastoma for a population of approximately 4 million. All charts

Table 19.3. *Medical problems of parents of 188 children diagnosed as having neuroblastoma between 1969 and 1986*

Maternal illness	Number of cases	Paternal illnesses	Number of cases
Manic depression	3	Diabetes	2
Anemia	3	Migraine	2
Chronic kidney illness	2	Hypothyroidism	1
Coronary disease	2	Reiter syndrome	1
Allergies	2	Erythema multiforme	1
Gastric ulcer	2	Pancreatitis	1
Migraine	2		
Carcinoma of cervix	2		
Leukemia (chemotherapy in pregnancy)	1		
Hypothyroidism	1		
Scoliosis	1		
Basal skin carcinoma	1		
Rheumatic fever	1		

were reviewed to ascertain the diagnosis by a report of pathological examination and to obtain details on maternal and paternal medical history.

In the reviewed period, 188 cases of childhood neuroblastoma were treated and available for review. In all of them, family history (negative or positive) was available, as summarized in Table 19.3. None of the mothers or fathers had had epilepsy or had been treated with phenytoin for other indications.

Statistical analysis reveals that, with the presence of no cases of phenytoin exposure in this cohort, not more than 1.5% of all neuroblastoma cases can be associated with such exposure (confidence limits of 95%).

Establishing the association between intrauterine drug exposure and postnatal cancer is of the utmost importance. Erroneous incrimination may be detrimental for women who need medications such as anticonvulsants.

Because of the rareness of virtually all childhood malignancies, case reports are the basis for determining causation of cancer. Such reports may be very useful in identifying drug-adverse effect associations when the drug and the adverse effect are both rare, because a small number of exposure-effect pairs may exceed by far the calculated chance of occurrence of the event. In that respect, the calculation by Ehrenbard and Chaganti[8] mentioned above is quite valid. The rate of occurrence of FHS is one in 5000 live births and that of neuroblastoma is one in 7100 live births[8]; therefore, it should take 35 million births for one case of both FHS and neuroblastoma to occur. These researchers calculated that it should take 45 years to have four such cases by chance in the United States, and not 5 years, as was the time between cases described until 1981.

That no further cases had been described until 1988 may reflect a reporting bias with clinicians not bothering to report additional cases of an "established" phenomenon. Alternatively, it may indicate that intrauterine exposure to phenytoin and neuroblastoma do not reflect a true association.

The five cases described in the literature are characterized not only by the child being exposed to phenytoin, but also being adversely affected by the FHS (Table 18.2). In the case reported by Allen *et al*[7], the mother had been on phenytoin since she was 5 years old, but her first three children were normal and only the fourth child had FHS and neuroblastoma. It has been postulated that the embryopathy seen in FHS is the result of the inability of some fetuses to hydrolyze the toxic arene oxide metabolite of phenytoin[9]. A study from our group has shown that the lymphocytes of children with major birth defects associated with FHS are unable to detoxify oxidative metabolites of phenytoin as well as do their peers not having FHS or having FHS and minor defects. Using this test, we did not detect abnormal detoxification by the cells of our index case with neuroblastoma. This suggests that the neuroblastoma may not be caused by or associated with an epoxide hydrolase deficiency. Conversely, the patient's brother, who has a clinical picture consistent with FHS, has an increase in toxicity to lymphocytes as does the mother. These results are in agreement with our previous reports that suggested that a human genetic defect in the detoxification of these metabolites exists in children with FHS and one of their parents[10].

Our index case did not have major anomalies consistent with FHS, and it is quite possible that an association between FHS and neuroblastoma does not hold true for the 90–95% of children exposed *in utero* to phenytoin but who do not suffer from FHS[12]. Of interest, the patient's half-brother, conceived by another father, has FHS and his mother was exposed to a relatively large dose of phenytoin; there are suggestions that FHS is more likely to occur at higher doses of phenytoin[13]. Because the metabolic deficiency postulated to cause phenytoin embryopathy (epoxide hydrolase deficiency) is rare (approximately 1 : 1000 are homozygous for this gene)[10], it is unlikely that both fathers of our patients are heterozygous for the gene, causing both the FHS and neuroblastoma to result from lack of epoxide hydrolase.

The rate of epilepsy in the general population in North America is 0.5%, and about half of these patients receive phenytoin[14]. Our serial cohort of 188 children with neuroblastoma, none of whom were exposed *in utero* to phenytoin, indicates that phenytoin cannot be incriminated in more than two cases of this series or in 1.5% of children in general with this malignancy.

In a recent case-control study examining drug risk factors associated with neuroblastoma in 104 cases, significantly elevated odds ratios were associated with maternal use of a neurally active drug in pregnancy, sex hormone exposure 3 months prior to or during pregnancy, frequent alcohol consumption during pregnancy, and maternal use of diuretic drugs during pregnancy[15]. These authors did not examine the association with antiepileptic drugs, but judging from the size of their cohort (about half of ours), it is unlikely that they had more than one or two such cases.

The results of our case study agree well with calculations based on available data from the United States. The Collaborative Perinatal Project reported on 132 cases of phenytoin use out of 50000 pregnant women prospectively collected[16]. The birth rate in the United States is 3 million per year; therefore, one would excpect 7860 pregnant users of phenytoin per year. Over 5 years, five cases of neuroblastoma asociated with phenytoin were described; therefore, the rate is one per 7860 cases of phenytoin, similar to that expected for neuroblastoma in the general population.

Using the same numbers, one would expect 786 cases of FHS per year in the United States if the rate of this syndrome is 10% of phenytoin users[12]. Consequently, one out of every 786 cases of FHS will have neuroblastoma, which is a tenfold increased risk compared with the general population. However, if one uses for the same calculation all the time period that has elapsed since the description of the association (1976–1988), then the relative risk for FHS being associated with neuroblastoma is not 10, but rather 4.2. Conversely, it is possible that the five cases of FHS reported in the literature are an underestimate of the US cases.

While our cohort does not have the statistical power to prove or reject an association between FHS and neuroblastoma, it suggests that intrauterine exposure to phenytoin cannot be considered as significantly associated with neuroblastoma in more than 1.5% of cases of the malignancy.

In utero carcinogenicity of cyclophosphamide

A variety of cancer chemotherapeutic agents have been shown to be carcinogenic in humans. Although potential fetal carcinogenesis caused by cancer chemotherapy has been mentioned as a possible adverse effect, no such reports have been published. We report on evidence of teratogenesis and carcinogenesis in a child following intrauterine exposure to cyclophos- phamide, whose twin sister was unaffected. Many of the major themes that are examined later in this chapter are illustrated by the following unique and remarkable case report. The case has been mentioned by us and others[17,18] and to the best of our knowledge is the only reported case of neoplasia following *in utero* exposure to chemotherapy.

The case description is followed by discussion of the known mechanisms of cyclophosphamide teratogenesis, available data on secondary cancer after this medication, and potential variabilities which may explain the different response of the two twins.

Case report

A gravida 3 para 4 29 year-old woman was diagnosed with acute lymphocytic leukemia (ALL) in February of 1968. Treatment was initiated with prednisone, 6-mercaptopurine (6-MP), and vincristine, resulting in a complete remission. The woman was maintained on vincristine and prednisone for 8 months. In November of 1968 she suffered a bone marrow relapse and was treated with aminoptherine, 6-MP, vincristine, and prednisone, again achieving remission.

In mid-December, the woman was started on a maintenance program of cyclophosphamide, 200 mg/day, with intermittent prednisone, both orally. Sometime in late December of 1968 the woman conceived and began to carry twins. The pregnancy was not discovered until August because of the woman's obesity and because she was amenorrheic.

The maintenance doses of cyclophosphamide and prednisone were continued until 4 weeks prior to delivery. In October of 1969, at 37 weeks' gestation, she had spontaneous rupture of the membranes and delivered male and female babies by vaginal delivery. The mother died of leukemia 21 months after giving birth.

According to the birth records from the delivering hospital, an apparently healthy girl weighing 1250 g and a boy weighing 1190 g were delivered. The boy had to be rotated from a transverse lie to a breech presentation with forceps. The girl also required forceps because she was in breech presentation.

While both babies were born with severe respiratory depression requiring intubation, the girl subsequently recovered and has since shown normal growth and development. At 9 years of age she had strabismus repair (September 1980) but has required no further hospitalization, and is 22 years old at present. She had her menarche at age 12 and has developed normal secondary sex characteristics.

The male child had multiple congenital anomalies severe enough that he required hospitalization until 10 months of age. He suffered from Madelung's deformity of the right arm, esophageal atresia, an abnormal inferior vena cava, and an abnormal renal collecting system later diagnosed as cross-renal atopia. The genitalia were normal, but the testes were not palpable.

After the second day of birth, a feeding gastrostomy was placed. In April of 1970, when the child was 5.5 months old, a primary anastamosis was carried out to correct the esophageal atresia. One month following this surgery, narrowing of the anastamosis site was found and required six dilatations over the following five months. During the surgery, an abnormality of the inferior vena cava was discovered. Eventually the child was felt to be well enough to be managed at home and was discharged in August of 1970.

Surgery was performed to correct the Madelung's deformity in March of 1971. At birth, hyperflexion of the wrist, marked right ulnar deviation, classical radial hemimilia, and an abnormal thumb were noted. Two unsuccessful attempts were made to correct the forearm deformity with plaster of paris casts. Therefore, the right radial club hand was centralized with a pin.

In November 1973, a number of tests were performed on the suspicion that the child suffered from Fanconi's anemia. Though the child had had severe anemia for the preceeeding two years, normal platelet, leukocyte, and reticulocyte counts, as well as genetic studies that found no evidence of increased chromosomal breakage, ruled out Fanconi's anemia. Chromosomal studies found 46 chromosomes of the normal male XY karyotype. There were no extra or missing chromosomes or abnormal banding patterns detected. A diagnosis of iron deficiency anemia was established and the child was treated with iron supplementation.

In 1976, the child was started on a long course of human chorionic gonadotropin (HCG) to descend the testes. While there was an increase in penile size and pubic hair, there was no change in testicular position. An orchiodopexy was performed in 1981 because of the failure of hormone therapy, at which time it was discovered that the left testicle was rudimentary and it was excised.

Serious developmental and neurological problems were diagnosed in 1978 when the local school board reported social and academic difficulties. A Wechsler intelligence test was performed when he was 11 years old showing the child to be in the low average range (full-scale IQ of 81), with verbal skills below this range.

On a number of occasions food became lodged in the esophagus. One of these occurrences led to the discovery of a hard thyroid nodule in the left and right lobes and isthmus in January of 1980. As well, enlarged cervical nodes in the neck were noted. A thyroid scan indicated a cold nodule, and following thyroidectomy the child was placed on thyroxine 0.1 mg/day. Pathological examination revealed papillary thyroid carcinoma. The father denied permission for further investigation.

A stage 3 neuroblastoma arising from the left adrenal gland necessitated immediate surgery due to rupture and hemorrhage in January 1983 when the boy was 14 years old. He received radiotherapy to the left upper abdomen totaling 3000 rad in 25 fractions over 5 weeks.

Two years later, a lymph node biopsy of the neck indicated metastatic papillary thyroid carcinoma. Thyroidectomy and modified neck dissection were carried out and a total of 350 mCi of I(131) was administered in 3 doses after 3 years to treat the primary cancer and two recurrences.

The most important question raised by this case is probably why two children who shared the same womb have such a dramatically different outcome. Previous studies have reported malformations due to exposure to alkylating agents (especially cyclophosphamide) in the first trimester. These malformations include absent toes, a single coronary artery, and umbilical and inguinal hernias[19–22].

The timing of fetal exposure to drugs and chemicals is critical to outcome. Exposure in the first trimester, during the period of organogenisis, may lead to gross congenital malformations and/or fetal death. Nicholson reported the incidence to be as high as 10% after first trimester exposure to cytotoxic agents[4]. Second and third trimester exposure may lead to retarded physical and/or mental growth and development, carcinogeneses, or infertility. These effects may not be apparent for a number of years[23].

To try to understand the differences in response between the twins, one should examine the mechanisms that may have contributed to their outcomes. It is unlikely that any complications experienced by the boy are the result of a twin pregnancy. Dizygotic (fraternal) twins are always diamnionic and dichorionic. Pregnancy complications occur less frequently in this group than in other twin pregnancies (for example, diamnionic monochorionic). In addition, these pregnancies usually go to term gestation[24,25].

The disparity between the twins may be the result of differences in their placentas' ability to metabolize cyclophosphamide. While it is known that the placenta has the ability to metabolize drugs[26], little, if any, research has been done to determine differences in the metabolic activity of twin placentas[27]. In the case of cyclophosphamide, the metabolites phosphoramide mustard and acrolein are more active than the parent compound[28,29].

Therefore, an increase in the metabolic activity of the boy's placenta relative to the girl's may explain the difference in outcome.

Cyclophosphamide is metabolized in the liver by cytochrome P-450 to 4-hydroxy cyclophosphamide (4-OHCP) which exists in equilibrium with aldophosphamide (Fig. 19.1).

Aldophosphamide undergoes spontaneous degradation catalyzed intracellularly by protein, cellular enzymes, and bases to form phosphoramide mustard and acrolein. 4-OHCP and phosphoramide mustard are cytotoxic *in vivo* and *in vitro*, but only the latter functions at physiological pH. Therefore, phosphoramide mustard is considered the ultimate alkylating agent. 4-OHCP and aldophosphamide can be oxidized to form inactive products by the enzyme aldehyde dehydrogenase, producing 4-ketocyclophosphamide and carboxyphyosphamide, respectively[28,29].

There is some dispute whether phosphoramide mustard or acrolein is the ultimate cause of teratogenicity[30–32]. Hales[30] injected phosphoramide mustard and acrolein into the amnionic fluid of pregnant rats. The malformations found in the fetuses produced by acrolein included forelimb and hindlimb defects, cleft palate, hydrocephaly, edema, and open eyes. In contrast, phosphoramide mustard produced only hydrocephaly, forelimb, and hindlimb defects.

The affected child may have been exposed to more active metabolites or intermediates than his sister if his placenta had a higher level of cytochrome P-450 activity. Alternatively, the girl's placenta may have protected her from some of the effects of the cyclophosphamide if she had a higher activity of aldehyde dehydrogenase. To date, no research has addressed the existence of polymorphism in placental metabolism of cyclophosphamide.

Another explanation may be differences in the hepatic cytochrome P-450 activity of the fetuses. In human fetal livers, drug-metabolizing activity has been demonstrated as early as 5–6 weeks of gestation, but there are considerable interindividual variations in activity levels[33,34]. An elevated P-450 activity in the boy could lead to increased formation of active intermediates and, therefore, greater exposure to the alkylating agents. Again, an increase in aldehyde dehydrogenase activity in the female could explain her normal outcome. It would be very interesting to be able to test both twins' cytochrome P-450 and aldehyde dehydrogenase levels, since differences present at birth may still persist 22 years later. However, the family declined any extra tests on the boy.

Cells may be protected from the effects of alkylating agents, including cyclophosphamide, by intracellular glutathione[28,30]. For example, the metabolite responsible for bladder toxicity in cancer patients has been

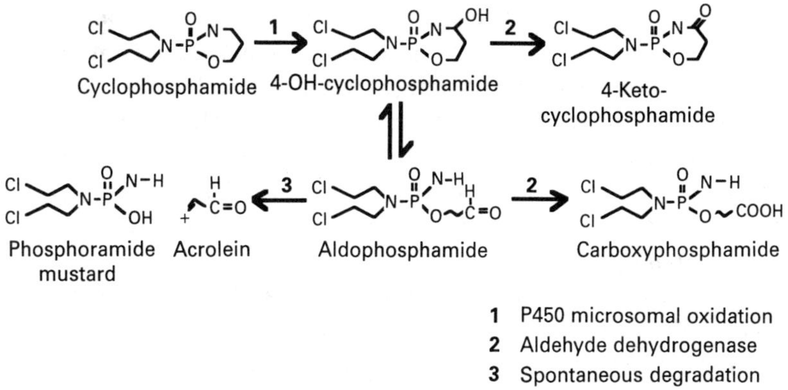

Fig. 19.1 The metabolism of cyclophosphamide.

demonstrated to be acrolein, and the administration of thiol compounds provides protection from bladder toxicity[30]. The presence of glutathione S-transferase has been found in fetuses[33], a deficiency of which in the male could have resulted in increased cytotoxicity. In addition, glutathione S-transferase is known to exist in the placenta[27], and differences in the levels in the two placentas may account for the variability in response.

Concomitant treatment with prednisone may have contributed to the deleterious effects on the boy. Faber *et al*[35] and Mouridsen *et al*[36] reported that prolonged treatment with 50 mg/day prednisone resulted in an increased rate of biotransformation of cyclophosphamide due to induction of cytochrome P-450. While induction of enzymes in the human fetus is thought not to occur until a few days before birth, placental enzyme activity has been induced by various agents[37].

The risk of second malignancies caused by alkylating agents, specifically cyclophosphamide, has been well documented[38–40]. Cases of bladder cancer, reticulum cell sarcoma, and acute leukemia have been reported by various authors[38,39,41]. It is plausible that the boy's cancers were second malignancies due to exposure to cyclophosphamide in the womb. Henne and Schmahl[42] documented the median time to appearance of solid tumors after exposure to cyclophosphamide as approximately 110 months. The latency period for the appearance of solid tumors among atomic bomb survivors was estimated to be 10 years[43]. These latent periods are consistent with the cancers in the boy occurring at 11 and 14 years after exposure to cyclophosphamide.

The increased risk of second malignancies due to alkylating agents of fetal DNA has been proposed elsewhere[44], but our case may be the first to be reported.

Because the long-term effects of chemotherapy are not always as clear-cut as in this case, it is reasonable to assume that a number of cases of growth and developmental delays, infertility, and cancer have occurred and have not been recognized. The first clinical transplacental human carcinogen, diethylstilbestrol also inflicts its effects more than a decade after exposure[2]. This means that much more effort may have to be focused towards longitudinal ascertainment of intrauterine exposures if we are to identify more such carcinogens.

With increased use of anticancer drugs for indications such as transplant and collagen diseases, it is likely that more fetuses will be exposed to these agents. More research is needed to elucidate mechanisms of teratogenicity and transplacental carcinogenicity of cancer chemotherapy.

References

1. Schuller HM: *Comparative Perinatal Carcinogenesis.* 1984, CRC Press, Boca Raton, Fla.
2. Herbst AL, Scully RE: Adenocarcinoma of the vagina in adolescence. A report of seven cases including six clear cell carcinomas. *N Engl J Med* 1971; 284: 878.
3. Ulfelder H: DES-transplacental teratogen and possible carcinogen, In: *Teratogen Update* (Sever JL, Brent RL, ed.) 1986; pp. 19–22, *AR Liss, Inc.,* NY.
4. Pendergass TW, Hanson JW: Fetal hydantoin syndrome and neuroblastoma. *Lancet* 1976; ii: 150.
5. Sherman S, Roizen N: Fetal hydantoin syndrome and neuroblastoma. *Lancet* 1976; 2: 517.
6. Ramilo J, Harris VJ: Neuroblastoma in a child with the hydantoin and fetal alcohol syndrome. The radiographic features. *Br J Radiol* 1979; 42: 993–5.
7. Allen RW, Ogden B, Bently FL, Jung AL: Fetal hydantoin syndrome, neuroblastoma, and hemorrhagic disease in a neonate. *JAMA* 1980; 244: 1464–5.
8. Ehrenbard LT, Chaganti RSK: Cancer in the fetal hydantoin syndrome. *Lancet* 1981; ii: 97.
9. Martz F, Failinger G III, Blake DA: Phenytoin teratogenesis: correlation between embryopathic effect and covalent binding of putative arene oxide metabolite in gestational tissues. *J Pharmacol Exp Ther* 1977; 203: 231–9.
10. Strickler SM, Donsky LV, Miller MA, Seni MH, Andermann E, Spielberg, SP: Genetic predisposition to phenytoin-induced birth defects. *Lancet* 1985; ii: 746–9.
11. Hanson JW, Myrianthopoulos NC, Harvey MAS, Smith SW: Risks to the offspring of women treated with hydantoin anticonvulsants with emphasis on the fetal hydantoin syndrome. *J Pediatr* 1982; 89: 662–8.
12. Briggs CG, Freeman RK, Yaffe SJ: *Drugs in Pregnancy and Lactation.* 1986; p. 353, Williams & Wilkins, Baltimore.
13. Yahr MD, Gudesblatt M, Cohen JA: Neurological complications of pregnancy. In: *Medical, Surgical and Gynecological Complications of*

Pregnancy. (Cherry SH, Berkowitz RL and Kasen G, eds.) 1961 p. 435, Williams & Wilkins, Baltimore.

14. Kramer S, Ward E, Meadows AT, Malone KE: Medical and drug risk factors associated with neuroblastoma: a case-control study. *J Natl Cancer Inst* 1987; 78: 797–804.

15. Heinonen OP, Slone D, Shapiro S: *Birth Defects and Drugs in Pregnancy*. Publishing Science Group, Littleton.

16. Shear NH, Speilberg SP: Anticonvulsant hypersensitivity syndrome: *in-vitro* assessment of risk. *J Clin Invest*, 1988.

17. Koren G, Demitrakoudis D, Weksberg R *et al*: Neuroblastoma after pre-natal exposure to phenytoin: cause and effect? *Teratology* 1989; 40: 157–62.

18. Reynoso EE, Shepherd FA, Messner HA, Farquharson HA, Garvey MB, Baker MA: Acute leukemia during pregnancy: the Toronto Leukemia Study Group experience with long-term follow-up of children exposed *in utero* to chemotherapeutic agents. *J Clin Oncol* 1987; 5(7): 1098–106.

19. Sokal JE, Lessmann EM: Effects of cancer chemotherapeutic agents on the human fetus. *JAMA* 1960; 172(16): 1765–72.

20. Nicholson HO: Cytotoxic drugs in pregnancy. *J Obstet Gynecol Br Commonw* 1968; 75: 307–12.

21. Greenberg LH, Tanaka KR: Congenital anomalies probably induced by cyclophosphamide. *JAMA* 1964; 188: 423–6.

22. Toledo TM, Harper RC, Moses RH: Fetal effects during cyclophosphamide and irradiation therapy. *Ann Intern Med* 1971; 74: 87–91.

23. Doll DC, Ringenberg S, Yarbro JW: Antineoplastic agents and pregnancy. *Semin Oncol* 1989; 16(5): 337–46.

24. Benirschke K: The placenta in twin gestation. *Clin Obstet Gynecol* 1990; 33(1): 18–31.

25. Johnson SF, Driscol SG: Twin placentation and its complications. *Semin Perinatol* 1986; 10(1): 9–13.

26. Van Petten GR, Hirsch GH, Cherrington AD: Drug-metabolizing activity of the human placenta. *Can J Biochem* 1968; 46: 1057–61.

27. Gottlieb K, Manchester DK: Twin study methodology and variability in xenobiotic placental metabolism. *Teratogenesis Carcinog Mutagen* 1986; 6(4): 253–63.

28. Moore MJ: Clinical pharmacokinetics of cyclophosphamide. *Clin Parmacokinet* 1991; 20(3): 194–208.

29. Jowett T, Wajidi MFF, Oxtoby E, Wolf CR: Mammalian genes expressed in *Drosophila*: a transgenic model for the study of mechanisms of chemical mutagenesis and metabolism. *EMBO J* 1991; 10(5): 1075–81.

30. Hales BF: Comparison of the mutagenicity and teratogenicity of cyclophosphamide and its active metabolates, 4-hydrocycyclophosphamide, phosphoramide mustard, and acrolein. *Cancer Res* 1982; 42: 3016–21.

31. Mirkes PE, Fantel AG, Greenaway JC, Shepeard TH: Teratogenicity of cyclophosphamide metabolites: phosporamide mustard, acrolein, and 4-ketocyclophosphamide in rat embryos cultured *in vitro*. *Toxicol Appl Pharmacol* 1981; 58: 322–30.

32. Spielmann H, Jacob-Muller U: Investigations on cyclophosphamide treatment during the pre-implantation period. II. *In vitro* studies on the effects of cyclophosphamide and its metabolites 4-OH-cyclophosphamide, phosphoramide mustard, and acroline on blastulation of four-cell and eight-cell mouse embryos and on their subsequent development during

204   *G. Koren*

implantation. *Teratology* 1981; 23: 7–13.

33. Wells, PG: Chemical teratogenesis. In *Principles of Medical Pharmacology*, (Kalant H, Roschlau WHE, eds.) 5th edn. 1989, pp. 650–653, BC Decker Inc., Burlington, ON.

34. Krauer B, Dayer P: Fetal drug metabolism and its possible clinical implications. *Clin Pharmacokinet* 1991; 21(1): 70–80.

35. Faber OK, Moursden HT, Skovsted L: The biotransformation of cyclophosphamide in man: influence of prednisone. *Acta Pharmacol Toxical* 1974; 35: 195–200.

36. Mouridsen HT, Faber O, Skovsted L: The metabolism of cyclophosphamide: dose dependency and the effect of long-term treatment with cyclophosphamide. *Cancer* 1976; 37: 665–70.

37. Rajchgot P, MacLeod SM: Perinatal pharmacology. In *Principles of Medical Pharmacology*, (Kalent H, Roschlau WHE, eds.) 5th edn. 1989, p. 692, Decker Inc., Burlington, ON.

38. Petru E, Schmahl D: Second malignancies – risk reduction. *Cancer Treat Rev* 1987; 14: 337–43.

39. Rieche K: Carcinogenicity of antineoplastic agents in man. *Cancer Treat Rev* 1984; 11: 39–67.

40. Tucker MA, Fraumeni JF: Treatment-related cancers after gynecologic malignancy. *Cancer* 1987; 60: 2117–22.

41. Coleman CN, Kaplan HS, Cox R, Varghese A *et al*: Leukemias, non-Hodgkin's lymphomas, and solid tumours in patients treated for Hodgkin's disease. *Cancer Surv* 1982; 1: 733–44.

42. Henne T, Schmahl D: Occurrence of second primary malignancies in man – a second look. *Cancer Treat Rev* 1985; 12: 77–94.

43. Beebe GW, Kato H, Land CE: Studies of the mortality of A-bomb survivors. Mortality and radiation dose, 1950–1974. *Radiat Res* 75: 138–201, 1978.

44. Willemse PHB, Van Der Sijde R, Sleijfer DT: Combination chemotherapy and radiation for Stage IV breast cancer during pregnancy. *Gynecol Oncol* 1990; 36: 281–4.

20
Fetal tumors

P. McPARLAND, G. RYAN AND D. FARINE

The inclusion of a chapter on fetal tumors in this book largely reflects the increasing detection over the past decade of "abnormal growths" during prenatal ultrasound. Tumors may be defined as local swellings from morbid or abnormal growth. The vast majority of fetal tumors are benign and can range from small lesions which may resolve, as in the case of some ovarian cysts, to aggressive, rapidly growing masses which, depending on their size and location, can be lethal or cause serious morbidity as occasionally seen with large sacrococcygeal tumors. Although there is an expanding body of literature on the subject, fetal tumors are rare and individual experience within any one unit is small. Before embarking on attempted treatment of a disease, it is imperative that the natural history of the disease be known. Unfortunately, termination of pregnancy and a variety of invasive techniques have often been performed without clear knowledge of the risk–benefit ratio. Acknowledging that these tumors are relatively rare, this chapter will attempt to discuss the incidence, pathology, natural history, ultrasonic appearance, differential diagnosis and management of tumors diagnosed *in utero*.

Teratoma

The most frequently diagnosed fetal tumor is a teratoma[1] and it is perhaps an exception to the above criticisms in that, because of its relative frequency when compared with other tumors, its natural history is reasonably well understood. A teratoma is a tumor of various tissues, chaotically arranged and usually of the most diverse types, with no relation to the site of origin. Cartilage, bone, epidermis, glandular epithelium, hair, teeth, etc. are common components, but other specialized tissues such as liver, kidney, nervous, eye and hematopoietic are also represented. Although rare in the fetus, because of their characteristic ultrasonographic appearance and thus their relatively easy diagnosis, they are well described *in utero*. They have been located in the spine, brain, head and neck and face and gonads most commonly. It is relevant to consider some of these separately as outcome is often dependent on location.

Sacrococcgeal teratoma

This is a tumor arising from totipotential embryonic cells of the coccyx. In the early embryonic period, an opacity formed by a thickened linear band of epiblast known as the primitive streak actively forms intraembryonic mesoderm until the end of the fourth week; thereafter, production of mesoderm and mesenchyme slows down. Normally, the primitive streak diminishes in size and gradually disappears. It is thought that, if remnants of the primitive streak/node persist, they give rise to a sacrococcygeal teratoma (SCT). Although reported as one of the commonest tumors in the neonate, the incidence of SCT is generally quoted as 1 in 35–40000. Females predominate over males with a ratio of 4 : 1, though the sex ratio in the incidence of malignant tumors is equal[2].

In the past the majority of cases remained asymptomatic *in utero* and were diagnosed after birth, but where routine prenatal ultrasound is employed they are being diagnosed increasingly when views of the spine to rule out neural tube defects are performed. They are also diagnosed when ultrasound is requested to aid management with polyhydramnios and in cases with elevated maternal serum alpha feto-protein. Most SCTs are solid or mixed with approximately 10–15% totally cystic, thus the diagnosis is relatively easy during a fetal anomaly scan. The presence of functioning choroid plexus, which produces CSF, is thought to be responsible for cystic components of the tumor. SCTs may be entirely external with a variable degree of pelvic extension, or the entire tumor may be in the pelvis with nothing visible externally. The American Academy of Pediatrics (AAP) has classified SCTs into four types: type I is predominantly exterior with only a minimal presacral component; type II is predominantly external, but with a significant intrapelvis component; type III is predominantly internal with type IV being entirely internal[3]. The external-type tumor accounts for 50% with only 10% being totally intrapelvic. In this AAP survey, 82% of all SCTs were benign with none of the type I tumors being malignant. The incidence of malignancy appears to be related to the age at diagnosis with few being malignant at birth but rising to 50% by four months of age.

The sonographic findings are of a mass arising from sacral and/or perineal region which is usually a mixed cystic/solid lesion. Although, as mentioned above, the diagnosis is relatively easy in the majority of cases, the 10% that are totally intrapelvic (type IV) may be missed. Associated findings include polyhydramnios which may be secondary to high output renal failure[4] or a transudation of fluid from the tumor; hydronephrosis secondary to lower urinary tract obstuction. The differential diagnosis of SCT is large and varied. It includes hydromyelia, chordoma, neurogenic tumor, liopma, rhabdomyoma sarcoma, extrarenal Wilm's tumor, hamartoma, neuroblastoma, hemangioma, malignant melanoma, ovarian and meconium pseudocyst. If the mass is cystic it may be confused with a myelomeningocoele. The latter is always associated with spinal dysraphism whilst, with an SCT, the posterior spinal anatomy is usually intact.

With the advent of antenatal ultrasound, the focus on SCT has shifted from management at birth to management in the antenatal period. A multidisciplinary approach involving the perinatologist, neonatologist and pediatric surgeon is optimal. The prenatal mortality differs from that seen postdelivery. Antenatal reports of SCTs suggest a mortality of 30–50%[5,6]. The commonest cause of perinatal loss is premature labor secondary to polyhydramnios. The development of hydrops and placentomegaly is a very ominous sign with a 100% (15/15) mortality in one series[7]. On this basis, fetal surgery with tumor resection has been advocated in selected cases if the hydrops appears before 28 weeks' gestation and the tumor is deemed respectable[8]. This approach seems reasonable but must be considered experimental. Because of the risk of dystocia and traumatic hemorrhage, cesarean section has been suggested if the tumor size is greater than 5 cm[9].

After birth, the outlook is largely determined by the size and location of the tumor. Complete excision of the tumor should be performed early in the neonatal period resulting in a favorable prognosis for those who survive surgery. Residual tumor may lead to malignant change and serial measurement of αfp levels may be useful. In general, surgery for types I–III is relatively easy and uncomplicated, though with large and vascular tumors, hemorrhage can be problematic. In this situation, some groups advocate preliminary transabdominal legation of the middle sacral artery. The mortality rises when diagnosis is delayed after birth. In a survey carried out by the Surgical Section of the American Academy of Pediatrics (AAPSS), there was a 7% mortality in 225 operated patients whose tumors were diagnosed at birth. This rose to 38% for these children who underwent surgery after 2 years. The recurrence risk of SCT is extremely low, though isolated cases have been reported.

Neck and craniofacial teratomas

These tumors are histologically the same as previously described. Most teratomas in the head and neck region are benign. Outcome depends on size and location. Intracranial tumors are often solid/cystic tumors that completely replace normal brain tissue. They account for approximately 50% of all congenital intracranial neoplasms. They may be benign or malignant, though both types, because of their location, carry a poor prognosis. Ultrasonically, these intracranial tumors can appear as large heterogenous disorganized masses with varied degrees of distorted cranial anatomy and, as such, are readily seen when axial views are taken, usually to measure the biparietal diameter which is an essential component of most prenatal scans. Commonly, obstructive ventriculomegaly is present and when the tumor mass is very large dystocia may occur. Most prenatal cases described in the literature result in perinatal demise[10] probably because these cases represent the large masses. Smaller lesions which may go undetected may have a good outcome if sited in a favorable location. Other intracranial masses which may resemble teratomas include medulloblastoma, epen-dymoma, choroid plexus papilloma, lipoma, astrocytoma and glioblastoma. If there is a substantial cystic component, the differential diagnosis would also include porencephaly and arachnoid cysts. Recently, it has been suggested that MRI scanning may improve the diagnosis of such masses.

Several hundred cases of neck teratomas have been described in the literature. Ultrasonically, these tumors are often well delineated due to anatomic encapsulation from surrounding tissue. The differential diagnosis includes cystic hygroma, sarcoma, haemangioma, thyroid goitre, branchial cleft cyst, neuroblastoma, laryngocoeles and thyroglossal cysts.

The prognosis is largely dependent on the size of the tumor. Small tumors are often easily respectable in the newborn period with good cosmetic outcome. Larger tumors are associated with respiratory obstruction and obviously require immediate surgery. Occasionally, with very large tumors, intubation may be difficult or impossible and death ensues shortly after birth. It may be appropriate in such cases to attempt intubation at cesarean section before delivering the body[11,12]. Such scenarios may be anticipated when prenatal ultrasound demonstrates hydramnios in association with an empty stomach.

The vast majority of these are identified at birth, though some are small and not easily seen. Tumors are usually unilateral, and located in the anterolateral aspect of the neck, but may cross the midline. In cases of large tumors, the fetal head may be hyperextended and/or laterally flexed during labor and cause dystocia requiring operative delivery (abdominal). Large tumors may also cause tracheal destruction[11]. Several cases requiring endotracheal intubation after delivery of the shoulders have been described, and antenatal detection of large or centrally placed tumors should alert to the possibility of difficult intubation.

In addition to the above sites, teratomas have been described in the placenta, umbilical cord, mediastinum, pericardium, liver and stomach.

The chest

By the second trimester, the pleural and pericardial cavities are morphologically distinct and the contents of these spaces are easy to visualize. It is routine at least to incorporate a cross-sectional view of the chest during a fetal morphology assessment. As a result, a variety of tumors involving the heart, lungs and pleura have been identified, but these tumors are extremely rare. The incidence of cardiac tumors at postmortem is 1 in 10000 at all ages and is thus much less *in utero*. The most common primary cardiac tumors in the fetus are rhabdomyomas which typically arise from the interventricular septum. These tumors are associated with tuberous sclerosis in 50 to 86% of cases[13]. Thus a careful clinical examination of both parents, specifically looking for cortical tubers, subependymal hamartomas, retinal hamartomas, adenoma sebaceum, evidence of mental retardation and other features of tuberous sclerosis is indicated. The size, number and location of rhabdomyomas vary. Their appearance is of a solid, echogenic mass located within the heart. The earliest diagnosis of rhabdomyoma was at 20 weeks[14]. They may be incidental findings during a routine scan or occasionally be diagnosed in association with hydrops. This may result from outlet obstruction or from a secondary supraventricular tachycardia as a result of accessory conductive pathways within the tumor. Once diagnosed, close fetal surveillance is indicated as rapid growth may occur both with both rhabdomyomas and teratomas leading to compromise when timely delivery may be beneficial if maturity allows. Depending on accessibility, such tumors can be removed after delivery with good outcome. Differential diagnosis includes teratoma, fibroma, myxoma, hemangioma and mesothelioma, which have all been described in infancy. A specific diagnosis is not possible prenatally, though multiple solid lesions are strongly suggestive of rhabdomyomas.

Masses that appear in the lung are usually developmental abnormalities (cystic adenomatoid malformations, bronchogenic cysts and extralobar sequestration) and not tumors and will not be discussed further.

The abdomen and pelvis

A vast range of abdominal and pelvic masses have been described prenatally. Only a minority would qualify as a tumor. They primarily concern the liver, kidneys, adrenal glands and ovaries. Hepatic tumors include hemangioma, teratoma, hepatoblastoma, hemangioendothelioma and rarely metastases from neuroblastomas. Hepatoblastoma is the most common hepatic malignancy in neonatal life, though only one fetal case has been reported. Its sonographic appearance is predominantly echogenic and may show areas of calcification. Hemangiomas have also been detected prenatally and contrast with hepatoblastoma in that their sonographic appearance is hypoechogenic. Several fetal deaths have been described with these tumors as a result of tumor rupture (either spontaneously or at delivery), compression of thoracic organs or hydrops secondary to arterio-venous shunting.

The kidney and adrenal glands

The most common type of renal neoplasm is mesoblastic nephroma. It affects males more than females. It is a solitary hamartoma usually with a benign course. The adjacent kidney is normal. The tumor does not have a well-defined capsule. Ultrasonically it appears as a large, solitary, predominantly solid, retroperitoneal mass arising from the kidney. Polyhydramnios is nearly always present, though the reason for this association is unclear. Its appearance may resemble focal renal dysplasia, teratoma, neuroblastoma of the adrenal and Wilm's tumor. However the latter is rarely seen before one month of age. Hydramnios may lead to premature labor. Unilateral nephrectomy after birth usually effects a cure.

After teratoma, one of the most commonly diagnosed tumors is adrenal neuroblastoma. This neoplasm is usually unilateral, though 50% have metastasized by birth. The most common sites for spread are the liver, subcutaneous tissue and placenta. The tumor appears as a unilateral growth of mixed solid and cystic texture located in the upper pole of the kidney. Fetal hydrops is often present. This tumor may be suspected when there is maternal nausea, vomiting and hypertension. These symptoms are caused by excessive production of catecholamines which cross the placenta. Perinatal management should include regular ultrasonic assessment of the mass. Consideration may be given to early delivery if rapid growth occurs.

The ovary

There are now several hundred cases of prenatally diagnosed ovarian cysts in the literature. These are generally small in size, but a minority may be so big as to cause dystocia. The prenatal diagnosis is based on finding an echo-free mass in the pelvis of a female fetus. The majority are benign cysts of germinal or graafian origin, such as simple cysts, theca-lutein cysts and corpus lutein cysts. Occasionally they may be septated as with theca lutein cysts. They are rarely seen before 30 weeks' gestation[15,16]. The differential diagnosis includes hydronephrosis, megacystis, meconium peritonitis, intestinal obstruction, duodenal atresia, choledochal cysts, hydrometrocolpos, and renal, urachal, duplication, omental and mesenteric cysts. The management of fetal ovarian masses is controversial. Serial ultrasound should be performed, as spontaneous resolution often occurs in the third trimester possibly secondary to the drop in gonadotrophins that occurs around term. Ovarian tumors may undergo torsion and hemorrhage *in utero*. Prenatal aspiration has been advocated in selected cases. The potential advantages include establishing ovarian etiology (analysis of aspirate cytology and biochemistry) and thus diagnosis; demonstrating the presence or absence of hemorrhage within a cyst and facilitating preservation of ovarian function both by reducing the risk of torsion and avoiding neonatal surgery[14]. Such an approach may be justified when the cyst is so large that pulmonary hypoplasia may ensue, or abdominal dystocia may result. There is less agreement on the role of aspiration in smaller cysts. Interestingly, there have been no cases of malignancy reported among ovarian cysts diagnosed prenatally. Over 50% undergo surgery in the neonatal period, though it is likely that a significant proportion could be managed more conservatively with spontaneous resolution[18].

Fetal metastasis of maternal tumors

The placenta serves as a barrier for metastatic spread between the mother and fetus. Even in widespread maternal metastatic disease there is almost never a spread to the fetal compartment. The converse is also true and the rare fetal malignant tumors do not affect any maternal organs. Potter and Schoeneman[19] reviewed all the iterature prior to 1970 and were able to find only 24 cases with maternal tumors spreading to the placenta. Only eight of these spread transplacentally to the fetus. These 24 cases included 11 cases of melanoma, 4 of breast carcinoma, two of stomach carcinoma, two of lung carcinoma and five of other single cases of other malignant tumors.

Seven of the eight cases with fetal involvement were melanomas. In a more recent review[20] there were 53 cases with metastic spread to the products of conception with 12 that metastatized to the fetus. More than half of these 12 cases were melanomas. This rate of melanomas is out of proportion to the frequency of melanomas which 8% of all malignancies in pregnancy. In contrast, breast and cervix carcinomas that account for more than half of the maternal metastic tumors had only eight reported cases of spread to the placenta and none to the fetus.

Conclusion

With the rapid progress of prenatal ultrasound, it is likely that, during the next decade, many more types of fetal tumor will be diagnosed during fetal life. This will help greatly in the diagnosis and early management of these conditions.

References

1. Werb P, Scurry J, Ostor A *et al*: Survey of congenital tumors in perinatal necropsies. *Pathology* 1992; 24: 247–53.
2. Ravitch MM: Sacroccoccygeal teratoma. In *Pediatric Surgery 2* (Ravitch MM *et al*, ed), 3rd edn. Chicago Year Book 1979.
3. Altman RP, Randolph JG, Lilly JR: Sacroccoccygeal teratoma. American Academy of Pediatrics Surgical Survey 1973. *J Pediatr Surg* 1974; 9: 389–98.
4. Bond SJ, Harrison MR, Schmidt KG *et al*: Death due to high-output cardiac failure in fetal sacrococcygeal teratoma. *J Pediatr Surg* 1990; 25(12): 1287–91.
5. Chervenak FA, Isaacson G, Touloukian R *et al*: Diagnosis and management of fetal teratomas. *Obstet Gynecol* 1985; 66: 666–71.
6. Sheth S, Nussbaum AR, Snaders RC *et al*: Prenatal diagnosis of sacroccoccygeal teratoma. Sonographic–pathologic correlation. *Radiology* 1988; 169: 131–6.
7. Harrison MR, Adzick NS, Flake AW: Prenatal management of the fetus with a correctable defeat. *In Ultrasonography in Obstetrics and Gynecology* 3rd edn. (Called, ed).
8. Langer JC, Harrison MR, Schmidt KG *et al*: Fetal hydrops and death from sacrococcygeal teratoma: rationale for fetal surgery. *Am J Obstet Gynecol* 1989; 160: 1145–50.
9. Gross SJ, Benzie RJ, Sermer M *et al*: Sacroccoccygeal teratoma. Prenatal diagnosis and management. *Am J Obstet Gynecol* 1987; 156: 393–6.
10. Ten-Brooke ED, Verdonk GW, Roumen FJ: Preantal ultrasound diagnosis of an intracranial teratoma influencing management: case report and review of the literature. *Eur J Obstet Gynecol Reprod Biol* 1992; 45(3): 210–14.
11. Langer JC, Tabb T, Thompson P, Paes BA, Caco CC: Management of prenatally diagnosed tracheal obstruction: access to the airway *in utero* prior to delivery. *Fetal Diag Ther* 1992; 7: 12–16.
12. Schulman SR, Jones BR, Slotnick N, Schwartz MZ: Fetal tracheal intubation with intact uteroplacental circulation. *Anesth Analg* 1993; 76(1): 197–9.

13. Harding CO: Incidence of tuberous sclerosis in patients with cardiac rhabdomyoma. *Am J Med Genet* 1990; 37: 443–6.
14. Groves AM, Fagg NL, Cook AC, Allan LD: Cardiac tumors in intrauterine life. *Arch Dis Child* 1992: 67 (10 Spec NO): 1189–92.
15. Rosenfield CR, Coln CD, Duenhoelter JH: Fetal cervical teratoma as a cause of polyhydramnios. *Pediatrics* 1979; 64: 176.
16. Rizzo N, Gabrielli S, Perolo A *et al*: Prenatal diagnosis and management of fetal ovarian cysts. *Prenat Diagn* 1989; 9: 97–103.
17. Meagher SE, Fisk NM, Boogert A, Russell P: Fetal ovarian cysts: diagnostic and therapeutic role for intrauterine aspiration. *Fetal Diagn Ther* 1993; 8: 195–9.
18. Muller-Leisse C, Bick U, Palussen K, Troger J, Zacharious Z, Holzgreve W, Schuhmacher R, Pantoja E, Llobot R, Gonzalez-Flores B: Retroperitoneal teratome: historical review. *J Urol* 1976; 115: 520.
19. Potter JF, Schoeneman M: Metastasis of maternal cancer to the placenta and fetus. *Cancer* 1970; 25:380.
20. Dildy GA, Moise KJ, Carpenter RJ, Kilma T: Maternal malignancy metastatic to the products of conception: A review. *Obstet Gynecol Surv.* 1989; 44:535.

Index